LIVING WITH OSTEOARTHRITIS

PATRICIA GILBERT trained at St George's Hospital Medical School, London, and worked in hospital and general practice in London and latterly for the Community Health Service in south Warwickshire. She was also the clinical tutor and visiting senior lecturer at Warwick University for a number of years. Writing is now a full-time occupation for Dr Gilbert, her most recent publications being *Helping Children Cope with Attention Deficit Disorder* (Sheldon Press) and a textbook for nursery nurses. She is married with two daughters.

Overcoming Common Problems Series

A full list of titles is available from Sheldon Press,
1 Marylebone Road, London NW1 4DU, and on our website at
www.sheldonpress.co.uk

Overcoming Common Problems Series

Overcoming Common Problems Series

Overcoming Common Problems

Living with Osteoarthritis

Dr Patricia Gilbert

sheldon PRESS

First published in Great Britain in 2003 by
Sheldon Press
1 Marylebone Road
London NW1 4DU

British Library Cataloguing-in-Publication Data

A catalogue record for this book is available from the British Library

ISBN 0–85969–887–4

1 3 5 7 9 10 8 6 4 2

Typeset by Deltatype Limited, Birkenhead, Merseyside
Printed in Great Britain by Biddles Ltd
www.biddles.co.uk

Contents

Acknowledgements

My thanks are due to the many people who have discussed with me the problems that they have experienced with osteoarthritis. Their personal difficulties have been of much value in – I hope – making this book helpful to the many others suffering from this common condition.

Especial thanks are due to Dr Mick Garratt, who devotedly read the text and came up with many useful suggestions from his own extensive experience.

This book is dedicated to the memory of my beloved husband, Victor, without whose help over many years my word-processing skills would have been negligible or non-existent.

Introduction

'Arthritis' is a term familiar to many in the older age group – and to a not insubstantial number of younger people. Arthritis can be thought of as a disease affecting one or more joints in the body, of which there are very many. Arthritis can, however, be due to over 200 conditions, all of which cause pain and other symptoms in the joints. The word 'arthritis' is often used to refer to any one of these conditions. For example, the disease rheumatoid arthritis is frequently confused with osteoarthritis. Both diseases cause joint pain, stiffness and immobility, but rheumatoid arthritis is an entirely different condition from osteoarthritis – the subject of this book.

In this book I have attempted to clarify the exact nature of osteoarthritis, which is a well-defined, specific medical condition. Possible causes, symptoms and signs, risk factors and different forms of treatment are discussed, along with basic descriptions of what actually happens to cause such pain, discomfort and disability.

I hope that readers will gain insight into these various aspects of osteoarthritis. It must be stressed, however, that for individual sufferers this book is no substitute for advice and diagnosis from a medical adviser. No book can ever replace the face-to-face discussion with a doctor, who, as well as listening, is able to see what is being described. But much can be done, by simple means, to reduce the disability so often encountered by people with this condition. Osteoarthritis, with its restrictions on daily living, is frequently accepted as just part of the ageing process. This is not necessarily so and living life to the full – even with osteoarthritis – should be a universal aim.

1

Osteoarthritis: an overview

Overall description of osteoarthritis

Osteoarthritis is just one of very many conditions that give rise to pain and discomfort in the joints of the body. These conditions are frequently called by the general term 'arthritis' and come under the wide heading of 'musculoskeletal disorders', so called because the affected part of the body is the bony skeleton and the attached muscles, which are necessary for movement.

Arthritis is a condition of the joints, which allow movement between the bones of the skeleton. Although '-itis' at the end of a medical word means 'inflammation', it is only in severe cases of osteoarthritis that inflammation plays a part. In fact, 'arthropathy', meaning simply 'disease of the joints', would be a more accurate term for what we call osteoarthritis. However, years of use of the word 'osteoarthritis' mean that everyone is aware of what is meant. Therefore 'osteoarthritis' is used throughout this book.

Some of the pain associated with arthritic disorders is due to spasm of muscles as they pull on the affected joint during movement. However, the main source of the pain arises from sensitive bone ends when they rub because the cartilage that normally protects them has been destroyed in arthritis.

Doctors who specialize in musculoskeletal disorders are known as rheumatologists. There is, of course – as with all branches of medicine – a good deal of overlap with other specialties such as orthopaedic surgeons and general physicians.

Musculoskeletal disorders are common, and it is thought that about 20 per cent of all visits to the doctor are due to some type of musculoskeletal problem. It is also estimated that up to 2,000,000 people in the UK have osteoarthritis to some degree. So it is a sizeable problem and one that accounts for much disability.

Osteoarthritic changes are seen in many vertebrate animals (i.e. animals with backbones). The joints affected vary in different types of animal. This is probably due to the specific stresses put on joints according to the main type of movement seen in each type of animal.

1

For example, the most commonly affected joint in horses is the hock, the backward-pointing joint in the hind leg. The most commonly affected joints in humans are the hip and the knee, with the joints of the fingers and thumb coming close behind. The elbow and the small joints of the foot also often become arthritic. Osteoarthritis can also occur in the spine, often following injury, typically a fracture caused by a fall or a sporting injury sustained many years previously.

Basic structure of joints

So what is so special about these joints that they should be so prone to osteoarthritis? Risk factors are discussed in detail in Chapter 4, but a look at the structure of affected joints can clarify the picture as to why it is that specific joints – hip and knee – often become arthritic.

The joints of the body are divided into a number of subgroups according to their specific structure and function. The knee and the hip are 'synovial' joints. They move freely, which is, of course, necessary so that walking can take place. The internal structure of these joints makes them prone to arthritic change. As an example, the ends of the bones making up the knee joint – the femur (thigh bone) and the tibia (shin bone) – are covered with thin cartilage. This cartilage is in turn covered with a specialized tissue known as the synovial membrane. This tissue secretes a fluid, the synovial fluid, that lubricates the joint in a similar way to the oil in the engine of a car. The whole joint is enclosed in a capsule of fibrous tissue, which links the two bones together (see Figure 1).

How osteoarthritis affects joints

It is when the cartilage of the joint becomes damaged that osteoarthritis occurs. Without the smooth surface of the cartilage protecting the ends of the bones they can rub together – painfully! The synovial membrane also becomes inflamed and secretes substances that further erode the cartilage and finally the bone itself (see Figure 2). When this happens the smooth functioning of the joint is affected, and pain and disability occur.

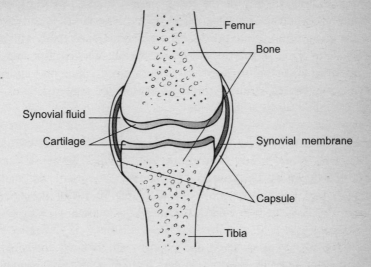

Figure 1 A normal knee joint

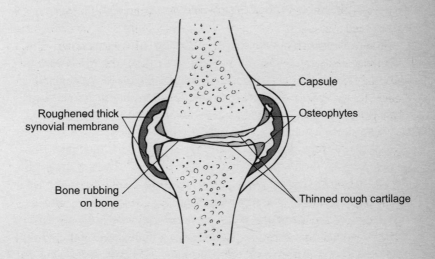

Figure 2 A knee joint affected by osteoarthritis

Osteoarthritis used to be thought of as a degenerative disease that progressed inexorably as the years passed because of the general 'wear and tear' of life. Today, however, osteoarthritis is considered to be more of an active process of destruction and repair. The processes involved in this to-and-fro condition are complex and are dependent on a number of extrinsic factors such as previous injury or being overweight. Basically in osteoarthritis, for some reason excess new bone is produced under the protective cartilage. This new bone eventually wears away the cartilage, and tiny fractures occur and extend down into the bony surfaces of the joint. The cartilage becomes irregular and eroded, owing to the actions of certain substances under the control of various enzymes. Inflammation occurs and this further thins the cartilage. In severe cases bony outgrowths occur, which further damage the smooth working of the joint and give rise to more pain and stiffness. If, however, the enzyme activity is reversed and changes are brought about in the substances that are causing damage to the joint, this somewhat gloomy picture can be halted. It is not known exactly why, or how, this process of healing and repair happens. It can be dependent on a number of factors, both inside the affected joint and outside it. The process of healing and repair is slow and occurs gradually over many months.

Certain factors are thought to help the healing process. For example, losing excess weight that the joint is having to support is one such factor. More complicated are the effects of rare genetic diseases that exert an influence on the degeneration of the cartilage of the joint. Previous injury that alters the structure of the joint, and therefore its function, can also play a part.

Recently, regular intake of cod liver oil has been thought to be involved in the destruction of enzymes that have adverse effect on the cartilage of synovial joints. More research on the reasons why this healing process occurs is under way.

It is strange, but true, that the same level of osteoarthritic changes – as seen with X-ray and other imaging techniques – causes different degrees of disability in different people. Not everyone with the obvious X-ray changes of osteoarthritis will have a similar amount of pain or stiffness. Therefore, it is important that careful clinical assessment is made for each individual patient regarding their disability, regardless of X-ray or other imaging changes.

While the hip and the knee are the two largest joints to be affected by osteoarthritis, other smaller joints of the body can also be involved. The small joints of the fingers are frequently affected in women around the time of the menopause. These small joints of the fingers become swollen and enlarged as the result of bony outgrowths. These bony outgrowths are known as 'Heberden's nodes', because they were described by Dr William Heberden in the late eighteenth century. They can give rise to difficulties in the fine movements of the fingers by causing stiffness and pain. Difficulty putting on or taking off a ring is often one of the first signs that a finger joint is beginning to be affected.

The joint of the thumb nearest to the wrist is also often affected by osteoarthritis. Initially the joint becomes swollen, inflamed and painful, and the joint can eventually become almost completely disorganized, with this part of the hand being markedly sunken inwards. This is known as 'Boucher's arthritis'. Activities such as unscrewing the lid of a jar can become virtually impossible, owing to loss or weakness of the grip between the thumb and the fingers.

Other sites of pain around a joint can be due to inflammation in a bursa, known as 'bursitis'. Bursas are fibrous sacs lined with synovial tissue. They are situated over protruding bony points of the skeleton and provide much-needed protection from everyday knocks and bumps. The two most common bursas to be affected are in front of the kneecap and on the outside of the big toe (causing a bunion). These bursas can become inflamed, usually because of excessive wear and tear, and can be exceedingly painful. (The bursitis affecting the knee used to be known as 'housemaid's knee' or 'clergyman's knee', owing to the time spent kneeling in these two occupations!) Bursitis can be acute and without treatment will become a chronic (long-term) condition – as anyone with a painful bunion will be aware.

Bursas are also found in other parts of the body – for example, in the shoulder, the elbow and the lower part of the pelvis. (Inflammation of the bursas in the pelvis used to be known as 'weaver's bottom'.) In the spine, particularly in the neck or the lower back region, the small bony protuberances that make up part of the spine's general structure can also be affected by osteoarthritis. Attached to these protuberances are strong muscle tendons, and therefore much pain and stiffness can occur on movement. (However, it must be remembered that there are many other conditions that can cause low back and neck pain. Osteoarthritis is just one reason for disability in these parts of the body.)

Possible causes of osteoarthritis

The above description briefly shows what is happening in individual joints. A broader overview of the possible causes of the problem needs now to be mentioned, i.e. the epidemiology of osteoarthritis – whom it affects and possible predisposing factors. (These will be looked at in greater detail in later chapters.)

Caucasian race

Osteoarthritis occurs in all populations of the world, although the joints affected do seem to differ from population to population. For example, osteoarthritis of the hip appears to affect South Asian and Chinese populations less than it does their Western (Caucasian) counterparts. Osteoarthritis of the hand is uncommon in Malaysian women.

Increasing age

Osteoarthritis can affect people under the age of 40, as can be shown on X-rays. However, these X-ray changes are frequently, although not always, without symptoms. As age advances the incidence of osteoarthritis increases – in those aged over 65, the incidence rises to over 80 per cent.

Female sex

Young men are more likely to suffer from osteoarthritis than young women, but over the age of 55 more women are affected. Why this is so is not completely understood, but differing hormones probably have a part to play.

Genetic inheritance

As with all our physical characteristics genetic inheritance plays a part in whether or not we shall suffer from osteoarthritis. Osteoarthritis is not a directly inherited characteristic, but there is certainly a strong tendency to osteoarthritis in some families. This is particularly evidenced by the onset of Heberden's nodes in women, where a strong familial tendency can be noted.

At-risk occupation

A person's occupation can have a marked effect on the development of osteoarthritis in later life. Men whose work involves a good deal of stooping or lifting of heavy weights are most at risk. Excessive sporting activity also has a part to play. Injuries of many kinds, whether due to sport or other forms of injury, are also a risk factor.

Obesity

Obesity seems to go together with the onset of osteoarthritis. It is difficult to decide, however, which comes first. Do people get osteoarthritis because they are overweight? Or are they overweight because they have osteoarthritis and so find movement difficult?

Summary

Whatever the potential cause, osteoarthritis is a common problem, especially during the latter years of life. Much pain and disability are experienced, together with many lost working days and lack of ability to enjoy the retirement years to the full.

2
Signs and symptoms of osteoarthritis

What is meant by 'signs' and 'symptoms'? 'Symptoms' can be defined as those subjective feelings associated with any disease process going on in the body. In other words how exactly the condition affects the life of the sufferer – the pain, discomfort and limitation to everyday life that are experienced. 'Signs' are the objective facets of disease. Signs may be able to be seen (either by eye or by imaging techniques), heard (as in a creaking joint) or felt (as in a swelling).

Much can be learned by sympathetic listening to someone describing his or her symptoms. A diagnosis can then be confirmed by a physical examination with further checks as may be thought necessary – for example, by blood tests or X-rays or other imaging techniques.

These definitions apply to any disease process in the body – but to get back to osteoarthritis . . . anyone with osteoarthritis will be able to describe exactly how it is affecting his or her life. The most usual problems experienced at first are pain and stiffness. These are closely followed by difficulty in movement, progressing finally to limitation of movement. Swelling around the affected joint or joints is a variable feature, as is the other common symptom, deformity of the joint. Let us look at these problems in more detail.

Pain

Pain in a joint is technically known as 'arthralgia'. It is important to determine exactly what type of pain is being felt, where the pain occurs, at what time of the day it is at its worst and if it is related to any specific activity.

Osteoarthritis is characterized by a gradual onset of pain in the affected joint, usually over several weeks or months. The pain does not arise suddenly in response to one specific movement; rather it slowly becomes obvious, particularly when a definite type of movement is undertaken. Many sufferers also say that the pain or discomfort becomes worse in certain adverse weather conditions, such as the damp, cold days of winter. This appears to be a subjective finding only (but one that is nevertheless very real to the sufferer) – there do not seem to be any obvious changes in the joint during these relatively short periods of time. However, it is a factor that causes much extra distress during winter.

If the pain is worse after a night's sleep or after some shorter period of rest during the day, it is probable that the joint is actively inflamed. Again this can be a variable problem, and there may be days or weeks when the pain is more severe before it decreases to a quieter level again.

Pain that suddenly becomes more severe needs to be taken seriously, and medical advice should be obtained. Such a happening is unusual in osteoarthritis, and infection in the joint may be the cause. The infective process will lead to an increase in the inflammation of the joint, with subsequent swelling caused by this inflammatory process. In severe cases of osteoarthritis in which the joint has been badly damaged by the disease process, a fracture can occur, and this will give rise to a similar sudden onset of pain. Likewise an alteration in the dynamics of the joint will give rise to a sudden increase in the severity of the pain, as Maureen's case history shows.

Maureen has suffered from severe osteoarthritis for many years. She has had a hip replacement and an elbow replacement over the past ten years or so. This has improved both her mobility and dexterity to a certain degree, but she is still not as spry as she would wish.

Having been a nurse all her life, Maureen knows the importance of avoiding excess weight. In fact, she has probably taken this to extremes, and she could be said to be too thin! But the years of lifting patients and being on her feet for many hours of the day have been undoubted factors in the onset of osteoarthritis in her later years. Although she had been looking forward to an active retirement, Maureen has been forced to accept that her physical limitations preclude many of the activities to which she had been looking forward for so long. During a particularly bad phase she was reduced to walking with two walking sticks around her one-floor apartment.

One unusually sunny day in an especially dull autumn, Elspeth, a friend and former nursing colleague, called to take Maureen out to lunch in the nearby town. Maureen enjoyed the brief car trip, since she now rarely ventures forth in her car. Elspeth parked as near as possible to the door of the restaurant, but there was still a walk of 100 yards or so.

'I can manage very well to walk,' Maureen insisted when Elspeth suggested that she drop her off and then go and park the car. 'I may be slow, but I get there in the end.' So the two walking sticks were rescued from the boot of the car, and Maureen and Elspeth set off down the street, Maureen leaning heavily on her walking aids.

'Why don't you try elbow crutches, Maureen?' suggested Elspeth as they wended their slow way along the road. 'I've been told that they are not suitable for my "tin" elbow,' replied Maureen as she carefully manoeuvred her way through the door of the restaurant, banging her arm sharply on the door jamb as she did so. 'Ouch!' she said under her breath, thinking how lucky it was that the elbow was the replacement one and not the other one. Being a stoical soul she did not mention the event to her friend. 'Kind people don't want someone who is always moaning,' she thought to herself.

Lunch was excellent, but Maureen ate only a little. Elspeth took no notice of this, being used to Maureen's small appetite, and remarking, yet again, how slim Maureen had kept over the years.

Later that evening Maureen found herself in a good deal of pain in her elbow and had to take a couple of the pain-killers that she had been prescribed. 'I wonder why this is so painful all of a sudden,' she mused. 'Perhaps it was walking so far on my sticks today. Oh dear! I am getting ancient!' She smiled wryly to herself.

Two days later she had to give in and admit that the pain had not subsided with rest and analgesics. Getting herself down to the surgery, after making an emergency appointment, was a harrowing business. She was glad to be able to sit down and rest awhile until her name was called.

Dr Barlow knew Maureen well, and realized that there must be something unusually wrong, and possibly serious, for Maureen to ask for help on an emergency basis. 'I think an X-ray of your elbow would be advisable. I'll get someone to take you round to X-ray straight away,' said Dr Barlow as she wrote out the X-ray request form. 'Are you sure you haven't knocked your elbow or stumbled and had to save yourself from falling in an awkward way?'

'Oh – well – yes, I remember now. I did knock this elbow the other day, but it was such a slight knock . . .' Maureen had not thought any more of the injury to that elbow a few days previously, but on explaining it to Dr Barlow it became clear to her that this could indeed have been the cause of her pain.

As suspected, the X-ray showed that the bone around the replaced elbow had been chipped, and this was undoubtedly the reason for the increased pain. Maureen's arm was immobilized in plaster, which together with an arm sling gave much relief. 'I should have known,' she told herself firmly, 'that any unusual severe pain, as I had, needs investigation.'

Site and type of pain

Many people can explain the exact site of their pain. If the pain is felt to be coming from inside the joint, it is probable that the joint itself is inflamed. On the other hand, pain that is felt around the joint is more likely to be arising from a spasm of the surrounding muscles. This spasm is due to the muscles attempting to protect the joint from movements that will cause pain. Muscles weakened by disuse can also be painful when an attempt is made to move the joint too vigorously.

According to personality, differing levels of pain are felt. Some stoical types will soldier on through severe pain whereas others will be in much distress. Anxiety and depression also play a part in the degree to which pain is experienced.

Stiffness

Stiffness around the affected joints is a common complaint in osteoarthritis. This is especially so when the larger weight-bearing joints are affected. All sufferers find that their stiffness is at its worst in the morning after a night's rest, and also, to a lesser extent, after shorter periods of inactivity during the day. This is due to the muscles surrounding and supporting a joint becoming stiff through temporary disuse. Unless these muscles are brought into use again by *gentle* exercise, the stiffness will persist and can become worse over time. However, with graded use, much of the stiffness wears off during the day. Moreover, without regular use, muscles can become wasted and so unable to fulfil their proper supportive and mobilizing functions. In severe arthritis, such muscles can be seen to be smaller and thinner. The joint itself will look large and swollen, and in large part this is due to the comparative smallness of the surrounding muscles giving this impression. This is why it is so important that good muscle tone should be maintained, as far as possible, in osteoarthritis.

Crepitus

Crepitus is the grating sound heard when two diseased bones rub together. It is a sign of severe osteoarthritis in the affected joint.

Limitation of movement

Limitation of movement is the obvious result of pain, stiffness and, eventually, muscle wasting. This in turn causes more pain as the smooth working of the joint is affected as it becomes stiffened and weak.

Deformity

When a joint becomes disorganized, deformity becomes obvious. Three further aspects that can add to this deformity are:

* swelling;
* bony outgrowths; and
* loose bodies in the joint.

Swelling

Swelling in the joint is due to the inflammatory process. When this inflammation occurs, fluid pours out from the synovial membrane inside the joint cavity. Along with this, the inflammation also causes warmth over the surface of the affected joint, and, sometimes, a generalized redness of the overlying skin. If the inflammation continues for some time, the synovial membrane itself becomes damaged and thickened. This then gives rise to permanent enlargement of the joint, with further deformity and limitation of movement.

Bony outgrowths

Bony outgrowths, known as 'osteophytes', can occur at the margins of a damaged joint and can add to the general visual deformity. This is often particularly in evidence in osteoarthritis of the fingers – the Heberden's nodes so frequently seen in the fingers of middle-aged and older women are bony outgrowths.

Loose bodies in the joint

In more severe cases parts of these bony outgrowths break off and are found free inside the joint capsule. They are then termed loose bodies. Loose bodies are most frequently seen in osteoarthritic knees. These loose bodies obviously give rise to further pain, limitation of movement and deformity.

Functional problems caused by osteoarthritis

When these changes occur in the larger weight-bearing joints, such as the hip or the knee, disability can be severe and can, at times, completely immobilize the sufferer, so that treatment becomes urgent.

Less functional disability occurs when the osteoarthritic process affects the fingers or the small joints of the foot. However, Heberden's nodes in the fingers and Boucher's nodes in the thumbs can also cause many problems related to normal everyday activities. Movements such as gripping or screwing or any activity that involves small, well-controlled movements of the hands (such as sewing or knitting) can be severely affected. In these circumstances, there are various aids to daily living that can be helpful (see Chapter 8).

Localized and generalized osteoarthritis

Osteoarthritis can be a localized or a generalized condition. The localized form, as the name implies, occurs when the disease process is confined to one joint, such as one knee or one hip. The generalized form is said to occur when there are three or more joints – or groups of joints, as in osteoarthritis of the fingers – involved. The generalized form can sometimes have a relatively sudden onset, and it can also be more severe in women than in men. Why this is so is not clear, but further research may well help to explain this difference.

Other causes of arthritis

It is important that osteoarthritis is distinguished from other conditions that can give rise to somewhat similar symptoms. These other conditions can be conveniently divided into:

- those that affect a single joint in the body;
- those that affect many joints in the body; and
- those that affect the major bony structure of the body, the spine.

Conditions that affect a single joint in the body

Gout
Gout has, rather unkindly, been laughingly connected entirely with high living or an excess of port. Although these things may have some slight bearing on the incidence of gout, it is certainly not the whole story. Gout is caused by the deposition of uric acid crystals in a joint, most commonly the big toe joint, the fingers or the elbows. Uric acid is found in the body as an end-product of the metabolism of substances known as purines. Normally a specific enzyme deals with this end-product so that any excess can be safely excreted from the body. In gout this enzyme process becomes deficient so that uric acid accumulates and finds its – uncomfortable – way into a joint.

Attacks of gout come on rapidly and are excruciatingly painful, so much so that at times bed clothes or normal clothing cannot be borne over the affected joint. The skin over the affected joint is red and shiny, and it can almost be seen to throb with the pain. The condition can occur completely out of the blue or it can be associated with bouts of infection somewhere else in the body. It can also follow a surgical procedure or, occasionally, the use of some drugs. Men are more commonly affected than women, and affected people are often overweight and have other gout sufferers in their family.

There are various drugs that can be used to treat gout.

Long-term 'gouty arthritis' can occur, and although there has recently been reported an increase in this form of arthritis, it is still comparatively rare. Confirmation of the origin of this long-term arthritis can be gleaned from the history of earlier attacks of gout and also from its specific X-ray appearances.

Other conditions caused by crystals

Other crystals can be deposited in joints and similarly give rise to arthritic changes. Calcium crystals are the most commonly found type of crystal after uric acid. Calcium crystal deposition mainly affects the knees of older women, and it can cause much pain, swelling and disability.

Septic arthritis

Septic arthritis occurs when a joint becomes infected with either a bacterium or a virus. Bacterial infection is the more common of the two. Older people are the most likely victims. Joints that have already been damaged by disease are usually affected, most commonly the hip and the knee. Pain is much in evidence, and often other general symptoms of infection (such as fever, fatigue and nausea) are also present. These general symptoms give important clues that infection is present and that it may be the cause of the acute joint pain.

There are a variety of ways in which infection can reach a joint:

- from injury;
- by direct spread from infection in a nearby part of the body; and
- by spread in the bloodstream from, for example, an abscess or an infected wound somewhere else in the body (this is probably the most usual route of infection and occurs especially in elderly people and in those who are having to take drugs that suppress the immune system for some other, unrelated condition).

It is important that appropriate treatment for septic arthritis and any underlying infection should be given rapidly.

Tuberculosis used to be a common cause of joint infection, particularly of the hip in children. This was to a large extent due to the drinking of unpasteurized milk.

Injury

It may seem unlikely that injury would be confused with osteoarthritis, but it is worth looking at a few specific forms of injury:

- sprains (because they are such a common injury); and
- tennis or golfer's elbow.

It is unlikely that a sprain, which is a comparatively mild albeit painful injury, will be confused with arthritis of any kind. A definite episode of trauma will be remembered, which is quite unlike the gradual onset of osteoarthritic pain. A sprain occurs when the tissues surrounding and supporting a joint are damaged. Common places for sprains are the ankle and the knee. With rest and general symptomatic treatment (possibly after an X-ray to exclude any possible fracture), a sprain will quickly heal, leaving no adverse after-effects.

Tennis or golfer's elbow occurs with overuse of the elbow in both these ball-centred sports. There can be many reasons why this happens, including lack of fitness and a less than perfect technique. Inflammation of the structures surrounding the joint is the cause of much of the pain, but it is probable that the joint itself also is inflamed. Rest, anti-inflammatory drugs and cooling dressings do much to limit the pain. Stretching and flexibility exercises will be needed at a later date to restore good function.

Frozen shoulder

Frozen shoulder is a condition with which many people are familiar. It is often thought of as being arthritic in origin, but this is not the case. Rather, it is due to an inflammation of the capsule of the joint, and it is acutely painful with much limitation of movement in the joint. It is not usually associated with any previous injury. Treatment with pain-killing drugs, rest and possibly an injection of cortisone into the joint eventually brings about a cure, although it may be some time before the shoulder can be moved with any degree of ease. When the acute pain has subsided, gentle stretching exercise should be a daily routine.

Plantar fasciitis

One further painful condition – this time of the foot – that needs a mention is plantar fasciitis. The thick fibrous tissue of the underside of the foot becomes inflamed at the point where it is attached to the bone (the 'enthesis'), and small painful nodules may also be present. Often plantar fasciitis occurs in people who have an unusual walking pattern or because of overuse or a mild anatomical abnormality.

Rest, with judicious padding to relieve pressure on the most painful part of the foot, together with correction of poor walking patterns or foot deformities if possible, do much to relieve this painful condition. Again, however, it may be some time before full relief is obtained. Ultrasound treatment can sometimes be of value in persistent problems.

Conditions that affect many joints in the body

Rheumatoid arthritis

It is not unusual for osteoarthritis and rheumatoid arthritis to become confused, especially when osteoarthritis affects more than one joint of the body. In reality the two conditions are completely different, the only common factor being painful joints.

Rheumatoid arthritis is an inflammatory disease that affects many joints of the body, together with inflammation of the surrounding tissues. The immune system plays a large part in the onset of this disease, as do genetic factors. As well as affecting joints, rheumatoid arthritis can also affect many other organs of the body. Women are slightly more at risk from this disease than men, and close family members of a person with rheumatoid arthritis are more likely to have the condition.

The joints of the hands, the wrists, the elbows, the shoulders as well as the ankles, the knees and the small joints of the feet can all be involved. (Unlike osteoarthritis, in which the hip is the most commonly involved joint, in rheumatoid arthritis the hip is less often involved at first, but it can become painful, as the disease progresses.)

Affected joints are swollen and painful, with marked deformity occurring relatively early. There are also frequently marked general systemic upsets at the onset of the disease with fever, fatigue and nausea playing an unpleasant part.

The aim of treatment is to relieve the pain, to prevent further deformity and to keep the person as mobile as possible. A variety of drugs are available, and gentle physiotherapy and exercise are also used in treatment.

Rheumatoid arthritis is a complex disease and further discussion of it lies outside the scope of this book. However, it must be stressed again that osteoarthritis and rheumatoid arthritis are two quite distinct diseases, although the two conditions do occur together in some people.

Psoriasis

Psoriasis is primarily a skin disease, but many people with the condition also have joints affected by arthritic changes. The arthritis of psoriasis can take a number of forms and can affect only one or a number of joints at the same time. The presence of the characteristic skin problems of psoriasis and specific blood tests can distinguish the arthritis of psoriasis from osteoarthritis.

Arthritis in viral infections

Viral infections such as rubella, some urinary infections and HIV (the virus that causes AIDS) can give rise to a form of inflammatory arthritis in many joints at the same time. Fortunately once the infection has been controlled as far as possible, the arthritic symptoms generally improve.

Polymyalgia rheumatica and fibromyalgia

Polymyalgia rheumatica and fibromyalgia can also mimic osteoarthritis. In both of these conditions the main problems are in fact in the tissues surrounding the joints.

Conditions that affect the spine

The spine is a marvellous piece of engineering and, considering the work that it has to do, it is incredible that it copes as well as it does. In addition to keeping the whole body upright and rigid, the spine has to allow for a variety of sideways, rotational and stretching movements. (Just look at any athlete and it can be seen how many differing movements are possible.) All of this is done by a number of specialized bones, the vertebrae, which are stacked up one on another and held in place by a system of ligaments and muscles. These ligaments and muscles help to maintain the normal spinal curves – as seen in the neck and lower back, for example. The whole structure is made flexible by spongy pieces of specialized cartilage between each vertebra, the intervertebral discs. These intervertebral discs also perform the vital function of being 'shock-absorbers' when, for example, each step is taken.

So, bearing in mind this basically unstable structure (dependent as it is on a number of anatomical features allowing for many different movements), pain in various parts of the back would seem to be more likely than not. Osteoarthritis can affect specifically the lower part of the back and the neck. It is the small 'winged' parts of the vertebrae that are affected.

Back pain can also be due to a wide variety of conditions other than osteoarthritis.

Prolapse of an intervertebral disc
Disc prolapse causes pain down the course of the nerve most closely associated with the involved intervertebral disc. Disc prolapse occurs most commonly in the lower part of the back, where it gives rise to the all too familiar pain of sciatica. Here it is the nerve pain that causes problems rather than the disease process in the spine. Severe cases of disc prolapse may need surgery.

Cancerous deposits in the spine
Cancerous deposits in the spine are, regretfully, an all too common cause of spinal pain. The actual primary cancer, which may or may not have been recognized, can be in any organ of the body. When the cancer spreads, via the bloodstream, to the spine, it can mimic arthritic pain. In these cases, the person will need treatment for the original cancer as well as relief for the bony pain in the spine.

Ankylosing spondylitis
Ankylosing spondylitis is a condition that affects movement in the lower part of the back. The bones of the vertebral column together with the sacroiliac joints are mainly involved. (The sacroiliac joints

are the joints between the lower part of the backbone – the sacrum – and the pelvic girdle, part of which is termed the ilium.) The onset is insidious with pain and stiffness after rest as the main symptoms, together with much fatigue. Improvement in stiffness is often seen after exercise.

Other parts of the skeleton are also often involved, notably the neck, the hips and the chest wall. Specific problems may also be seen in the eyes, the lungs and the bowel.

Treatment is pain relief and exercises that are designed to strengthen muscles; swimming is especially beneficial. Good postural habits are also important.

Summary

Many conditions can affect the joints and bones of the body. It can be difficult at times to determine the exact cause of pain, stiffness and immobility. Osteoarthritis tends to be blamed for many musculoskeletal problems, but it is important to remember that there are other conditions that give rise to pain, stiffness and immobility. Therefore, it must be stressed that medical advice must always be sought for any long-term or severe joint pain.

3

Investigations and assessment

As with all disease processes, the ultimate diagnosis of osteoarthritis, with its typical features of pain, stiffness and immobility, is made by a number of well-defined steps. First, the history – the symptoms actually felt by the sufferer – is important. This will begin to eliminate other possible causes of the pain and other associated symptoms.

Second comes the clinical examination of the affected part of the body.

Third comes confirmation of what has already been discovered – with the diagnosis strongly suspected – by X-ray or other imaging techniques.

Finally comes the assessment of the amount of disability caused by the condition. For example, how is everyday life affected? Is work being made difficult or even impossible?

The patient's history

The history from the patient of any disease is the linchpin of diagnosis. By asking relevant questions, the doctor can narrow down the likely diagnosis to a relatively few possibilities. In addition, the patient and doctor will become acquainted, learn to understand what each is trying to convey and, most important of all, establish a trusting rapport. This is of prime importance in a potentially long-standing rheumatic disease such as osteoarthritis. Treatment and advice on how best to improve life over the succeeding years must be the common aim of the patient and the doctor. Much more can be achieved by working together than from the sum of all the various interventions that may be necessary. Getting on the same wavelength is the initial, vital part of this process.

As a starting point, descriptions of the type of pain, where it is felt to be at its worst and how long the symptoms have been present all need to be confirmed.

Type of pain

Pain can be difficult to describe, but usually joint pain is described as a dull, continuous ache. The pain from nearby muscles and ligaments, which can also be affected, may give rise to sharp twinges. The pain from trapped nerves in the neck or lower back are often described as tingling pains – or, as one patient described it 'as if my arm were being pushed into a prickly hedge'.

Position of the pain

As we have seen, osteoarthritis affects synovial joints. It can be confined to one joint, such as the hip or the knee, or it can be more widespread and involve both these joints, together with the smaller joints of the hand or foot. Sorting out where exactly the pain is felt gives valuable clues to the diagnosis.

Pain is not always felt most severely over the affected joint. For example, pain may be felt in the knee even though it is the hip on the same side of the body that is in fact affected by osteoarthritis. Similarly, pain felt down the leg and into the foot can be due to problems in the lower part of the back; in this case a 'slipped disc' pressing on a nerve emerging from the spinal cord gives rise to this distant pain. Or again, pain felt in the upper arm can be due to problems in the shoulder joint.

Extra clues as to the cause of the pain can be gleaned by any associated symptoms in a specific joint. An example of this is the red-hot swelling of a joint affected by gout or other crystal deposits. Knees in a severe inflammatory stage of osteoarthritis can also be swollen as well as being acutely painful.

Timing of the onset of pain

Pain and stiffness due to osteoarthritis will have been noticed to be coming on over many months or even years. This is in direct contrast to the pain of an injury, the pain due to an acute onset of rheumatoid arthritis or the pain following a previous generalized illness that has led to a transitory inflammatory type of arthritis.

Important clues can also be gained from the duration of the symptoms. Constant bone pain that is not relieved by rest, exercise or the usual pain-killing drugs can be a sinister sign of a possible malignant cause. Pain of this type prevents sleep, which is rare in osteoarthritis except in very severe disorganization of a joint.

The pain of an inflammatory arthritis, including an acute inflammatory stage of osteoarthritis, is at its worst in the mornings. The pain then gradually improves over the course of the day, perhaps because of gentle exercise or the use of an anti-inflammatory drug. At a later stage of the condition, if severe joint damage has occurred, pain will be experienced to a greater degree as the day progresses when the joint is in constant use.

Other symptoms associated with the pain

Stiffness

Stiffness is an extremely common complaint in osteoarthritis. It is most noticeable on getting up in the morning. A long period of rest during the day can also give rise to this unpleasant symptom. In uncomplicated osteoarthritis, stiffness should improve within an hour of starting normal activity in the morning or after a rest. In an inflammatory phase of osteoarthritis and in arthritis due to any other inflammatory process, the stiffness will take longer to wear off.

Swelling

Swelling of an affected joint is not unusual. Two factors can be involved:

- an inflamed synovial membrane; or
- bony outgrowths.

An inflamed synovial membrane can cause joint swelling, which can at times progress to more swelling as more and more fluid exudes into the joint cavity. On occasions the swollen area can feel hot to the touch if an inflammatory process is the cause. This can be extremely uncomfortable and cause a good deal of limitation of movement.

Swellings can also be due to bony outgrowths ('osteophytes'). If so, the swelling comes on gradually and, after an initial period of pain, usually becomes less painful. A good example of this is the Heberden's nodes that are found on the fingers. These nodes may look unsightly and cause difficulties with dexterity, but at least they have the advantage of being relatively painless.

There is a specific swelling known as a Baker's cyst, which arises at the back of the knee. This swelling is filled with synovial fluid and results from either a tear in the capsule or over-production of synovial fluid in the knee joint.

Locking

Locking is a further symptom, which applies specifically to a knee joint affected by osteoarthritis. It is due to bony outgrowths that become detached and float freely in the joint as loose bodies. These loose bodies at times get into such a position as to fix – or lock – the joint into one, painful, position. These loose bodies require surgery if the locking becomes too frequent or painful.

General, non-specific symptoms

Any recent general symptoms, such as tiredness, weight loss, fever, rash or general feelings of lassitude, are also important. With this information, conditions such as systemic lupus erythematosus, Lyme disease and gonorrhoea, which can cause arthritic symptoms, can be excluded. Psoriasis, which is primarily a skin disease, can also cause arthritis, as can some forms of inflammatory bowel disease. Fortunately these conditions are relatively rare and there will be other symptoms, besides the arthritis, more in evidence.

Disability

The amount of disability caused by the arthritis needs to be fully checked out. Is it possible, for example, for normal day-to-day activities such as dressing and bathing to be done? Is climbing stairs proving difficult or impossible? And how about the general household tasks that need to be done on a regular basis – again, are these difficult or impossible?

It is also important to think about what help is available. For example, is a partner, or other nearby friend, involved in helping with everyday tasks?

Employment and sporting history

Finally, questions need to be asked about present or previous employment, which may be a factor in the onset of osteoarthritis. For example, labourers involved in heavy work on building sites, and farmers, are more prone to osteoarthritis in the joints that are involved in these types of work – the knees and the hips.

Previous sporting activities, such as contact sports and gymnastics in which there is much pressure on weight-bearing joints, can be a forerunner to osteoarthritis in later life. Dancers, too, are especially prone to arthritis in the small joints of the foot, owing to the excessive strain put on these small joints over a long period of time.

Previous injury, whether due to accident or surgery on a joint, can also predispose to arthritis at a later date. Operation on the cartilage around or in the knee is a good example of a possible previous cause of present osteoarthritis.

All of these enquiries will give valuable clues to the exact cause of the pain, stiffness and disability. It is vitally important that all other possible causes of the joint pain are excluded. A good history, as outlined above, is an excellent starting point.

Examination

A full clinical examination of the musculoskeletal system is time-consuming since there are so many anatomical structures involved. Bones, joints, muscles, ligaments and tendons, with their connecting blood vessels and nerves, all contribute to the smooth pain-free movement of the skeleton. Fortunately, a full examination of all these structures is often unnecessary. Quick screening tests will show where the major problem is, and a more detailed examination of the affected part can then follow. A common system of clinical screening is termed by the acronym 'GALS'. This abbreviation – so beloved of medicine – refers to the examination of movement of specific parts of the body:

G – Gait
A – Arms
L – Legs
S – Spine

By running through this check, the doctor can identify the part of the body that is most affected.

Gait

Gait plays an important part in everyday life. The smooth, fluid walking, running and jumping gait that is seen in youth can be quickly upset by any disease of the musculoskeletal system. Walking consists of smooth rhythmical movements of the legs in sequence, but arm movements in rhythm with each step are also involved. (Watch someone walk away from you – you will be surprised at just how much arm movement is involved. Notice, too, the interruption in the smooth flow of the gait in older people.)

Pain in any of the joints involved in walking – hip, knee or spine – will destroy fluidity of movement. This, at its worst, can result in an obvious limp, but a slightly uneven gait can result from muscle spasm around a painful joint.

Stiffness can also be recognized by an unevenness in the length of the stride on the affected side of the body. It is usually easy to see which hip is affected by the small step taken on this side. The side on which the walking stick is used can also give valuable clues, the stick being used to support the affected, weakened limb.

Arms

Looking at outstretched arms can reveal any obvious swelling or deformity. For example, in osteoarthritis of the thumb joint, the usual rounded eminence at the base of the thumb is lost, giving the joint a sunken appearance. Muscle wasting, resulting from disorganization of the joint, is the cause of this.

Approximating each finger in turn on to the pad of the thumb on the same hand demonstrates whether there is any loss of smooth movement. In rheumatoid arthritis, this movement can be especially difficult and there is also tenderness over the joints of the hands. This finding is not marked in osteoarthritis. In osteoarthritis of the fingers there may be obvious swelling of affected joints and limitation of movement but with comparatively little associated pain. Gripping an outstretched finger also gives valuable clues as to the strength of hand and finger muscles. Any pain or weakness associated with this movement – as is found in rheumatoid arthritis – will also be obvious. Limitation in any of these simple tests will be reflected in the performance of everyday activities such as gripping the lids of jars (so firmly fixed these days!), performing screwing motions or firmly grasping handles of cooking utensils. Other daily aspects of living can readily be thought of.

Placing the hands behind the head will show up any pain or lack of movement in the shoulder joints.

These quick initial tests on the arms can show any need for further detailed examination of the joints involved in each specific movement.

Legs

A lot of information about any involvement of the legs will already have been gained by the observation of the gait. Further examination of the knees and hips can localize any suspected problem.

It is easiest for the doctor to examine the hip and knee joints with the patient lying flat on the back. All movements of both hips and knees can then be assessed, together with the visual impact of any swelling or obvious deformity. As a joint is moved gently into various positions, crepitus (a creaking sound caused by the rubbing of tissues inside a joint) can be both heard and felt by an examining hand in severe osteoarthritis. The range of movement of both these major joints can be found by specific, passive positioning of the leg while the patient is lying on the back.

Active movements of the ankle can demonstrate problems in the small joints of the foot. If these joints are involved they will probably be tender when pressed, and this will, of course, be obvious when the patient walks.

Spine

Two distinct parts of the spine need to be examined in the quest for osteoarthritic changes – the neck (the cervical spine) and the lower back (the lumbar spine).

Neck pain can be due to a number of conditions, ranging from an acute spasm of the neck muscles to the degenerative changes of osteoarthritis. Other reasons for neck pain include:

• injuries to the neck, such as a whiplash injury following a road traffic accident;
• infection;
• malignant changes due to disease elsewhere in the body; and

- poor working conditions, for example when typing or reading.

The formation of bony outgrowths ('osteophytes') in the neck can also give rise to symptoms of dizziness and faintness, owing to pressure on the vertebral arteries, which pass up in the back of the neck close to the spine on their way to the brain. Degenerative changes caused by osteoarthritis are frequently found in the neck in people aged over 40, but often there are no symptoms despite obvious X-ray changes.

Lower back pain is common. Over 80 per cent of the population suffers from it at some time during their lives. Lower back problems are the cause of much pain, discomfort and loss of working time. Causes are legion and include:

- a 'slipped' disc (prolapsed intervertebral disc);
- degenerative changes in the three small joints between each of the vertebrae, and if osteophytes are present, weakness or tingling feelings in the legs can occur as well as pain;
- ankylosing spondylitis, a generalized disease in which lower back pain is much in evidence;
- malignant changes secondary to cancer elsewhere in the body;
- spinal stenosis, which occurs when the passage through the backbone in which the spinal cord rests becomes narrowed because of degenerative disease;
- referred pain from another disease in the abdomen, such as an abdominal aortic aneurysm (a 'ballooning' of the aorta, the main artery in the body); and
- poor posture, which is probably the most common cause of all, and includes poor positioning during the working day – the best example of this probably being long hours spent with a bent back when working at a computer keyboard.

X-rays and other imaging techniques

Confirmation of the diagnosis is then sometimes required by imaging techniques, which can show the extent and degree of osteoarthritic changes. These techniques include:

- plain (ordinary) X-rays;

- computed tomography (CT) scanning;
- magnetic resonance imaging (MRI);
- ultrasound; and
- isotope scanning.

Of course, not all of these investigations are necessary in every individual case. Each technique is useful in a variety of ways. Some are especially helpful in unravelling conditions that affect bone, others are useful in diseases of cartilage and the soft tissues surrounding a joint, while others highlight conditions inside joints.

Plain X-rays

Plain X-rays are most often the first line of investigation. This imaging technique is of value for:

- determining any narrowing of the space in between the bones of a joint – this is useful in the investigation of hip problems;
- discovering the presence of osteophytes;
- noting the presence, and extent, of fluid in a joint (known as 'effusions');
- finding osteoporosis (thinning of the bone) – this is especially common in post-menopausal women, and is a large subject on its own; and
- discovering the presence of any cysts in the joint.

One disadvantage of plain X-ray imagining is that, with the exception of septic arthritis, the disease process has to be fairly well advanced before any X-ray changes can be seen. Serial X-rays of the same joint taken over a period of months or years will show the deterioration – if any – that has taken place over time. However, this is of less value in osteoarthritis than in another common disease of bone, osteoporosis.

Ultrasound

Ultrasound has a few specialized uses:

- showing any loose bodies in the joint; and
- the size of a joint effusion.

CT scanning

CT scanning is useful for providing detailed information on the state of the bone. For example, it can detect the presence of osteophytes and any excess calcification of the bone. Three-dimensional views can be obtained by the use of specific computer software.

MRI

MRI has advantages over CT scanning. It provides a better image of the soft tissues surrounding joints, ligaments, tendons, intervertebral discs and muscles. The beautifully clear views seen on MRI are comparable to an excellent anatomical drawing.

Other imaging techniques

Other specialized techniques are also available for particular problems. For example, isotope scanning is used to pin-point:

- any secondary cancerous deposits in bone;
- any severe infective disorder in bones or joints.

Contrast arthrography uses a contrast medium, which is injected into the joint before a CT scan is done, to look for loose bodies or to show up small fractures or tears within the joint.

These relatively recent imaging techniques, and others, have vastly improved the diagnostic tools available for the investigation of all rheumatic diseases.

Other investigations

Two further procedures need to be mentioned in the investigation possibilities of osteoarthritis. 'Keyhole' diagnosis is performed by passing an optical instrument into a joint (usually the knee). This technique is termed 'arthroscopy', and it can also be used to perform surgical procedures within the joint cavity.

Second, fluid can be removed from a joint (again most frequently the knee) with a syringe. This will relieve the tension – and the pain – inside the joint as well as allowing the fluid to be checked for infection.

Note that blood tests give very little information about osteoarthritis. Only the absence of rheumatoid factor is of value in distinguishing osteoarthritis from rheumatoid arthritis.

Assessment of disability

Following on from these investigations comes the important assessment of just how much the disease is affecting everyday life. Questions need to be asked about aspects such as:

- the ability to walk any distance without having to stop because of increased pain;
- whether stiffness is affecting the ability to walk, and also at what time of the day any difficulty caused by stiffness is at its worst;
- the ability to climb stairs – is this difficult? impossible?;
- the ability to carry any weighty objects such as shopping (weakness caused by a lack of muscle tone will make this chore difficult, particularly if the lower back is involved);
- the ability to enjoy a good night's sleep – pain from severe arthritis or cancerous deposits in the bones will have a marked effect on sleep;
- the ability to dress, and if there are difficulties, whether it is the larger items of clothing or the buttons and other fastenings that are proving difficult – the smaller items can be difficult if fingers are involved;
- whether joints 'lock', so making movement of the joint impossible;
- whether the pain is generalized all over the body – if so, this could point to fibromyalgia being a sole, or added, problem;
- how much independent living is being lost and whether daily tasks are being achieved at all or perhaps only partially; and
- whether social activities are being curtailed?

These questions, and others relevant to each individual patient, will give a good idea of the amount of the disability being caused by osteoarthritis. From this, a plan of treatment can be suggested.

4
Risk factors

There are several factors that are known to be associated with the onset of osteoarthritis. Some of these are quite beyond our control, but others can be modified. (It must be remembered, however, that not all osteoarthritis diagnosed positively on X-ray or other imaging will inevitably cause pain and disability. It has been said that as many as 50 per cent of people with X-ray signs of osteoarthritis have no symptoms at all. Nevertheless, the remaining 50 per cent are a sizeable number of people, and some of these people have debilitating symptoms.)

Unmodifiable events

Genetic predisposition

Apart from choosing our parents – an impossible task! – there is absolutely nothing that can be done about genetic predisposition to osteoarthritis, which does seem to be a potent factor in whether a person will develop the condition.

There have been various studies on this subject. Probably the best known is the study of identical twins carried out in London in the 1990s. This research looked at identical twins (who have the same genetic inheritance because they arise from the same fertilized ovum) and non-identical twins (who have a different genetic inheritance). It found that an identical twin was more at risk of developing osteoarthritis if the other twin had the condition than a non-identical twin was.

It has also been found that 20 per cent of people with significant osteoarthritis have other family members suffering from the same condition, although different parts of the body may be affected. This is especially in evidence in women with Heberden's nodes, the typical swellings on the joints of the fingers. If your sister has Heberden's nodes, you too, if you are female, are three times more likely than average to be affected in the same way (see Bethany's case history).

Recent research has isolated the gene, or group of genes, responsible for the occurrence of osteoarthritis. The basic cartilaginous defect is now known to be the inherited factor. This is a major advance and could well be the basis of gene therapy for the future prevention and treatment of osteoarthritis. An exciting prospect.

'I hope I don't get bumpy fingers like Aunt Margaret when I get old,' 12-year-old Bethany whispered to her mother as she watched her great-aunt stitching away carefully at a hem that needed turning up.

'I heard that, Bethany,' smiled Aunt Margaret as she reached for the scissors. Little did young Bethany know just how much she too disliked the look of her hands, which, once upon a time, had been slender and beautiful. And how much it cost not to wince as she painfully manipulated the scissors with her arthritic thumb. 'You may never have hands like mine – your mother hasn't. Nor painful knees,' she added under her breath.

Genetic inheritance can play complex tricks. Although Aunt Margaret had osteoarthritis of her fingers (Heberden's nodes, as Bethany was to learn later in life) and osteoarthritis of her knees, Bethany's mother's generation seems to have missed out on this painful aspect of age altogether: Bethany's mother is now 75 years old and has no sign at all of osteoarthritis. However, Bethany herself, in her fifties, already has the beginnings of osteoarthritis in two of the fingers of her right hand. They were red and swollen a few weeks ago but have now settled into a quiescent state, nevertheless with the 'bumpy fingers' of her now long-dead great-aunt.

'And to think I was rude about Aunt Margaret's fingers.' Bethany smiled to herself as she remembered those bygone days, getting carefully and painfully to her feet rubbing her knees as she did so.

Generations can indeed be missed, but being female Bethany always stood a greater chance than her brother of knowing the pangs of osteoarthritis in later life. He, a healthy 50-year-old, still plays competitive sport with no seeming disability at all. 'Life never was fair,' commented Bethany.

Sex

Being female, and especially if you have other family members suffering from osteoarthritis, is not good news! The incidence of osteoarthritis in the hands, knees and small joints of the foot is greater in women than in men in the older age group (those older than 55 years of age).

On the other hand, mild arthritis in larger joints seems to affect both men and women equally. As age advances, however, there is a marked increase in the number of women being severely affected.

It has been suggested that female sex hormones have a bearing on this difference in incidence. Some studies have shown a reduced rate in the occurrence of osteoarthritis in women receiving hormone replacement therapy (HRT) at, or around, the menopause. This would confirm the importance of hormonal influence in the onset of osteoarthritis.

Age

As is obvious from what has been said above, age certainly plays a part in the onset of osteoarthritis. However, do remember that osteoarthritis is *not* an inevitable part of the ageing process. There are many other significant factors involved. It may be that previous injury or a deficiency in the repair mechanism of articular cartilage can also play a part as the years pass.

Osteoarthritis that is causing symptoms is uncommon in people under the age of 45 years. Below this age, men are more likely to be affected by the troublesome effects of osteoarthritis. It is thought that as many as 80 per cent of people aged over 65, both men and women, have osteoarthritic changes visible on X-ray. However, not all of these people have any symptoms. After this age, other factors, such as general health, physical fitness and ability to exercise, determine the amount of disability.

Race

Osteoarthritis occurs in people of all races. It appears not to be influenced by ethnic origin, climate or geographical location. (Cold weather does seem to play a part in the amount of pain and stiffness felt by those people with existing osteoarthritis. Why this is so is not clear, but anyone with osteoarthritis will be certain that it really is so.)

The pattern of disease varies, however, in different races. For example, osteoarthritis of the hip is less common in Asian races than in Caucasian races. Osteoarthritis of the hand, so common in women in the Western world, is rarely found in African women.

Other medical conditions

Other diseases, as has already been seen, can also give rise to arthritic changes. Psoriasis is just one such example, and other rare diseases such as acromegaly and haemochromatosis can also have associated arthritis.

Other problems in the soft tissue surrounding joints, such as occurs in fibromyalgia, plantar fasciitis or bursitis, can fudge judgement as to how much disability is due to osteoarthritis and how much to the other disorder. Similarly gout and septic arthritis, for example, need to be recognized and treated before all symptoms are laid at the door of osteoarthritis.

In some conditions that cause hypermobility of joints, osteoarthritis can be a later manifestation, probably caused by the extra stress put on the joints by the excessive movement.

Rheumatoid arthritis sufferers can also have extra problems if osteoarthritis becomes an added burden to their already damaged joints.

Some congenital deformities, which may be unnoticed in earlier life, can also lead to arthritis in later life.

It is important that any of these diseases are recognized and adequately treated as well as attention being paid to the osteoarthritis.

Modifiable events

Obesity

Obesity is the most important modifiable factor associated with the onset of painful osteoarthritis. Although it does not actually cause arthritis, excess weight adversely affects the progression of the disease. Just think of the extra strain on already diseased and underachieving joints, such as the hips and knees, that a stone or two of extra weight can impose! Well worth trying to slim down!

It has been suggested that a controlled and sustained loss of weight, if you are overweight, can halve the rate of progression of the disease. But just what is thought of as an ideal weight for someone approaching middle age? Apart from those people whose weight is necessarily controlled for their occupation – film stars, sports personalities – we all gain a few pounds as we mature. A good rule of thumb is that we should weigh no more than 9.5 kg ($\frac{1}{2}$ stone) more than we did at 21 years of age.

Middle-aged people do seem to be more at risk of severe symptoms of osteoarthritis than older people. This may be due to the relative 'slimming down' that occurs in old age, or it may be because middle age is a time when a more active lifestyle is sought, and so the symptoms associated with osteoarthritis exert a seemingly greater effect.

In a well-known study undertaken in the 1950s, a strong association was found between being overweight and the onset of osteoarthritis of the knee 36 years later. So it would appear that keeping a check on weight when relatively young is an important factor in achieving a relatively pain-free old age.

Occupation and sports

There have been no well-conducted studies to determine whether or not occupation has an effect on the onset of osteoarthritis in later life. There is good subjective evidence, however, that work that involves a good deal of bending, either at the hips or at the knees, increases the likelihood of later problems. Farmers and labourers, who often have to do a lot of bending together with lifting heavy objects, are examples of those most at risk because of their occupation.

Dancers, physical education teachers and people who take part in weight-bearing sports have also been found to have a probable higher risk of developing osteoarthritis of the hips and knees later in life. (In contrast to this, though, long-distance runners and track sprinters do not appear to be as susceptible as other people partaking in weight-bearing sports.) It is to be hoped that modern training methods, with the help of up-to-date equipment and an awareness of the potential problems, may help to reduce the association between certain sports and osteoarthritis.

Previous injury

A joint that has been previously injured has a higher potential to develop osteoarthritis. Even if the joint itself has not been directly involved in the injury, a break or injury to an adjacent bone can exert an effect on the nearby joint. For example, a severe break of an ankle, with the need for long-term immobilization of the leg, can put a strain on hips having to cope with an altered distribution of weight. Fractures that actually involve a joint will also obviously give rise to a greater risk of later osteoarthritis, owing to the episode of disorganization of the joint that resulted from the fracture.

Similarly, any previous operation on a joint can be a further potential cause of osteoarthritis. This is seen frequently in operations to repair a damaged ligament inside or on the outer aspect of the knee, a problem that occurs most often in knee injuries sustained during contact sports.

Previous injury cannot truly be said to be a modifiable factor, but it is as well to be aware of future possibilities.

Summary

The chances of developing osteoarthritis in later life are largely beyond our control. Being able to choose one's genes, sex, race – and age – is a pipe dream. Choosing one's occupation and avoiding injury would be the next most useful option. But the one aspect that is in our control is avoidance of excessive weight. Diet forms a large part of weight control. A complete re-think of eating patterns is often needed to maintain an ideal weight, and a less sedentary lifestyle is also helpful.

5

Treatment (1): how to help yourself

Before we discuss self-help ways of coping with osteoarthritis, a few words about the actual aim of any form of treatment may be useful. It may seem ridiculous to ask what is the aim if treatment when laid low with a potentially long-term disease such as arthritis. Life should be lived to the full, even with osteoarthritis. There are many ways in which this can be made possible – by self-help, by other ways that do not involve drugs or surgery and, finally, by prescribable drugs or surgery. At present there is no definitive cure for osteoarthritis, so all treatment needs to be aimed at preventing the condition from worsening as well as at relieving painful symptoms.

This chapter and Chapters 6 and 7 discuss the methods of achieving these aims. It must be remembered, however, that a positive diagnosis of osteoarthritis is vital, since embarking on treatment for osteoarthritis without being sure that it is really osteoarthritis that is causing the symptoms could cause more harm than good. So accurate medical diagnosis is a very necessary first step. (Remember, too, that should symptoms worsen – either rapidly or over a few weeks – medical advice will again be necessary to be sure that a further disease process is not intervening.)

Although, for ease of understanding, treatment has been divided into three chapters, all methods of help appropriate to each individual patient need to be considered. For example, one or two aspects from the self-help treatments together with one item, perhaps physiotherapy, from the non-drug group may work wonders. For someone else, prescribable drugs together with one or two self-help measures may be the way forward.

Remember also that it is the 'whole' person that needs to be treated and not just specific aspects of the disease. We are all individuals and what suits one person will not necessarily have the same good effect on someone else. A holistic approach that looks at all aspects of individual personality, lifestyle and expected future prospects is necessary.

Weight control

Weight control is probably one of the most helpful ways in which anyone can assist in relieving the symptoms of osteoarthritis. All of us gain some weight over the years and we can never expect to regain the slim sylph-like figures of youth. A little extra weight (up to, say 9.5 kg or $\frac{1}{2}$ stone on top of our weight when we were 21) has only a small effect. It is a gradual piling on of the pounds over the years that can become a serious problem. General health can suffer, and the extra weight puts an immense amount of strain on joints leading to a worsening of an incipient osteoarthritis.

Much has been written on the best way to control excess weight gain. Many people try the 'miracle' weight-loss regimes that abound. Care needs to be taken with the most extreme of these. Weight can indeed be lost rapidly. If this is done, however, at the expense of adequate nutrition, further health problems will occur. (Perhaps the most extreme example of this was someone whose diet was exclusively restricted to carrot juice. Weight was certainly lost, but at the expense of health and eventually of life itself.) Moreover, if weight is lost too rapidly, it can return just as quickly once the restrictive diet ends and the person returns to a more normal eating pattern.

So how can weight be kept under control? Two main ways are the cornerstones of weight control – diet and exercise.

Diet

Foods can conveniently be divided into four main groups:

- protein;
- fat;
- carbohydrate; and
- vitamins, minerals and trace elements.

Our food also contains a certain amount of fibre and roughage.

Protein

Protein is essential for healthy living. The building blocks of protein, amino acids, are the very stuff of life itself. There are 20 of these amino acids, but just 9 of them are 'essential' – meaning that the body will not remain in health if any 1 of these 9 is not included regularly in the daily diet. Without adequate daily protein intake the body loses its ability to repair tissues of all kinds that are affected by the general 'wear and tear' of daily living.

First-class protein is found in meat, fish, poultry, cheese and eggs. Second-class protein is available in pulses such as nuts, beans, peas, lentils and soya. Vegetarian diets, which exclude some of the first-class proteins, need to be carefully controlled so that sufficient other protein foods are taken in daily. A vegan diet, in which no first-class protein is taken at all, needs special care (see also the section on vitamins below).

Fat
Fat can be obtained from both animal and vegetable sources. Animal fat includes that found in meat and in dairy products such as cheese and butter. Vegetable sources of fat include the polyunsaturated oils (found in corn and sunflower oil and, to a lesser extent, plant sources). A certain amount of fat is necessary in a balanced diet, but excess intake of this type of food will, of course, add to the problems of increased weight.

Carbohydrate
Carbohydrates provide 'instant' energy and are vital as part of a healthy, controlled diet. Carbohydrates are found in bread, potatoes, pasta and rice. This food group forms the basis of many dishes.

Vitamins, minerals and trace elements
All of these substances are necessary for health and must be taken in adequate quantities on a daily basis. A good mixed diet will automatically contain enough of these substances. Frequently, however, the diet of older people is not adequate from this viewpoint – and, of course, it is older people who suffer most frequently from osteoarthritis. So, for some people, vitamin and mineral supplements are advisable. (Strict vegans are deficient in vitamin B_{12}, a vitamin that is necessary for the production of blood, among other needs. In these circumstances this vitamin will need to be given by injection on a regular basis.)

Minerals such as iron, calcium, potassium and magnesium are also vital for good health. Iron is necessary for healthy blood formation, calcium for healthy strong bones, potassium for strong muscles and normal heart rhythms, and magnesium for maintenance of healthy connective tissues.

Other trace elements, in tiny quantities only, are necessary – selenium and zinc are two of these. They will be present in adequate quantities in any good mixed diet.

A dietary supplement, glucosamine, has been found by many people to be helpful in controlling the symptoms of osteoarthritis. This seems to act helpfully on the damaged cartilage in joints. No definitive clinical trials have as yet been carried out on glucosamine, but there would seem to be no adverse effects reported at present from the regular use of this substance in the suggested amounts.

Fibre and roughage
Although they are not definite food products on their own, fibre and roughage must be part of a healthy diet. They are found in wholemeal bread, cereal, fruit and vegetables of all kinds.

Practical dietary advice
You musn't forget, when setting out on a diet to control weight, to incorporate all these food types into your daily diet. Without going into detail about a sensible diet (which is outside the scope of this book) a few pointers will help you towards a steady weight loss that can also be maintained. This may mean a different way of eating from what you have practised for perhaps many years. So be prepared for a different look to the shopping list! Remember:

- reduce the amount of fat in your diet (use semi-skimmed milk, remove all fat from meat, reduce the amount of butter or margarine you eat and restrict your intake of hard cheese) and fats high in polyunsaturates need to be high on the list of consumed fats;
- never fry food – grill instead;
- stay away from all sweets and chocolates, except for the occasional treat;
- eat fresh fruit instead of stodgy sweet puddings;
- avoid 'snacking' – so no biscuits or cake with your mid-morning

or afternoon drink – eat three adequate meals a day with only drinks (preferably water) if needed at other times to allay thirst (this can also help to allay hunger pangs);

- white meat or fish is preferable to red meat, which can contain excess fat, and oily fish such as mackerel, tuna and pilchards, which contain omega-3 oil, are thought to have a beneficial effect on the damaged cartilage of joints, helping with the repair process; and
- use low-fat salad dressings and low-fat yoghurt.

In addition to these possible changes in your dietary pattern, remember to:

- eat smaller portions at each meal – try using a smaller plate as a well-filled smaller plate is preferable psychologically to a half-empty large one; and
- weigh yourself weekly – the aim should be to lose 1–1.5 kg (2–3 pounds) steadily every week until your ideal weight is reached.

The next problem will be keeping to this weight. It is all too easy to slip into bad eating habits again – holidays and festivals are particularly dangerous for this! Obviously a little relaxation is allowable once your target weight has been gained, but you may need to reassess your eating habits after a few months. Perhaps a return of osteoarthritic symptoms will show the need for this.

There have been many articles and books written claiming miraculous cures of arthritis with specific diets. There has been a lot of scientific research into any connection between diet and arthritis. No positive results have been obtained, except that a healthy well-balanced diet will generally improve health as well as controlling weight.

Once you have achieved a reasonable weight for your body build and age, the next cornerstone – exercise – will be more easily undertaken, and even perhaps enjoyed!

Exercise

Exercise may well be the last activity osteoarthritis sufferers feel they need, but still more serious disability can arise from lack of exercise. It can easily be thought that exercise will 'wear out' damaged joints. However, as we have seen, 'wear and tear' is not the whole story in osteoarthritis; rather is it a cycle of damage and repair. Without exercise muscles become weaker and less able to protect the joint that they surround.

Exercise of itself – even without the added benefit of helping weight control – is beneficial for arthritis sufferers. There are three main physical advantages:

- strengthening and improving the tone of muscles – joints are protected more efficiently by good muscular strength and tone;
- suppleness – by putting joints through their full range of movements on a daily basis, flexibility is better maintained, although obviously movement of damaged joints needs to be limited at first and no movement that causes excessive pain should be done (stop as soon as pain becomes a problem);
- stamina, which is the strengthening of many body organs – heart and lung function, for example – can be improved by graded exercise and, following on from this, tissues will be better oxygenated by the improved blood flow.

Without exercise:

- the range of movement in the affected joints is decreased through disuse;
- balance can be directly affected, owing to the loss of muscle strength, leading to an imbalance in various joints and also to an increase in the risk of having damaging falls;
- production of synovial fluid, the 'oil' of the joints, can be diminished; and
- general fitness declines and psychological factors can become more of a feature – for example, it can be very easy to slip into a depressive state if general feelings of ill health as well as symptoms of osteoarthritis are present every day.

Walking
One of the best exercises, needing no special equipment except a comfortable pair of shoes, is walking. A daily walk, slowly at first and for a limited distance, will increase muscle strength, improve general stamina (making the heart and lungs work with greater efficiency) as well as increasing the flexibility of many joints. If you

have not been in the habit of walking you may feel some extra stiffness and pain in the muscles initially. However, with perseverance and a gradually increasing distance, much benefit will be noticed. If arthritic pain is especially bad on one day, limit your exercise and, of course, if excessive pain in damaged joints occurs, take a good long rest period.

Do not expect the pounds to drop off rapidly just because you are walking each day, but remember that the walking will be going along with your new, healthier diet. (Be careful, therefore, not to give in too often to a cup of hot chocolate and a cream cake when your walking brings you home with a healthy appetite!)

Swimming

Another excellent exercise that is enjoyable as well as being beneficial is swimming. The buoyancy of the water on the body will lessen the strain put on arthritic joints while still allowing a full range of movements in the hips, knees and shoulders. It will also increase stamina. Again, an excessive length of time swimming should be avoided at first – it is amazing just how tiring 15 minutes' swimming can be. But with practice the length of time can be increased, with added benefits. A swim twice a week, if possible, should be the aim.

Cycling

Cycling too is a good exercise. Joints are moved in a regular rhythm without excessive weight being transmitted through these joints. Leg and back muscles are strengthened by cycling, and it also helps to improve the suppleness of joints. Be sure that your bicycle is the correct size for your height or joints will not gain the full benefit. When sitting on the saddle it should be possible to touch the ground with your toe.

Care needs to be taken, however, on today's busy roads, particularly if muscles are relatively weak so that quick movements are difficult. A cycle track where cars and pedestrians do not need to be considered is ideal if one can be found locally.

Other forms of exercise

As well as general exercise in the form of walking, swimming or cycling – or even gentle gardening within the limits of kneeling, bending and so on – there are specific aerobic exercises that can be done to improve your strength, suppleness and stamina. ('Aerobic' exercises are those that increase the pulse rate and make you mildly breathless.) Obviously these need to be graded over the weeks and months and should never be done if there is any degree of discomfort. By gradually increasing the type and number of exercises, you can increase the stamina of your heart and lungs, which will benefit your whole body. Remember the importance of gentle 'warming-up' and 'cooling-down' exercises at the beginning and end of an exercise session.

Physiotherapists can advise on suitable exercises for each individual arthritis sufferer, and there are any number of books available that explain these exercises. 'Exercise and Arthritis', a leaflet from the Arthritis Research Campaign (see page 81), is a good source of information.

Aquarobics, exercises that are done in water, are excellent. The water allows movements to be done with greater ease. Exercising with other people, especially those with similar difficulties to yours, can be fun as well as beneficial.

Yoga is a good way to improve both strength and suppleness. The specific movements performed slowly and gently also help with breath control. A good teacher will be able to advise which exercises can be helpful for each specific disability and can also advise which movements should not be practised. An example of exercises to be avoided would be the exercises involving kneeling for a person with arthritic knees. Once the movements have been learnt, practice can continue at home.

The relaxation periods practised at the beginning and end of yoga sessions are also valuable in reducing tension. Tension can play a part in the amount of pain experienced. Tense muscles go into spasm and so increase pain. Relaxation techniques are all part of yoga programmes.

T'ai chi is a technique of gentle rhythmic exercise that can help to strengthen muscles and improve balance. Co-ordination is also improved as muscles become stronger. Initial classes are necessary to learn the specific movements. These can then be practised at home if classes are infrequent or difficult to attend.

Osteoarthritis is a condition in which immobility is to be avoided at all costs. Joints that are not exercised on a regular basis will

48

become stiffer. This will increase the pain as well as reducing the efficiency of the re-lubrication of the joint caused by the improved blood supply that comes about with exercise. Exercises suitable for each individual sufferer can be found, and can certainly delay the worsening of the disease and even in many cases reduce the severity of the symptoms. However, exercise, whilst generally toning up the body, will not of itself quickly reduce weight. The two prongs of attack need to be both weight control and exercise.

Keeping generally fit

These activities – weight control and exercise – will improve general fitness as well as improving the arthritic problem. Keeping generally fit is an important part of self-help for any disease. Obviously this can vary with each specific condition, but osteoarthritis is a condition in which fitness of both mind and body can vastly improve life.

Sleep

As part of the fitness programme it is important that a good night's sleep is made part of the 24-hour routine. Pain can make sleep difficult. Taking a pain-killing drug half an hour before bedtime with a hot drink (not a stimulant such as tea or coffee) will increase the possibility of getting off to sleep. To give yourself the best chance of getting a good night's sleep, try:

- to have a routine of going to bed and getting up each day at the same time;
- to avoid stimulating drinks, conversations or TV or radio programmes before going to bed;
- to have a bed that is firm and comfortable;
- to avoid a stuffy bedroom – open a window unless the weather is too severe;
- to resist firmly the temptation to get up to make a cup of tea, do the ironing or read the paper if you find sleep impossible – by doing this a habit will soon be formed, so instead make a conscious attempt to relax tight muscles one by one.

If sleep is still elusive remember that relaxation of the body alone without actually falling asleep is an important factor in refreshment for the next day's activities.

Mental attitude

Remember too that as well as looking after bodily fitness it is important to have a positive attitude. Many osteoarthritis sufferers become depressed about their condition. Life is difficult, morale is low and interest in outside activities is minimal. These feelings, understandable as they may be, only serve to increase pain and inactivity, so a vicious circle is set up. Hard as it may seem at first, taking gentle exercise and finding a (perhaps completely new) hobby will do much to make pain more bearable.

Remember that most people with osteoarthritis do not become severely disabled. Rather, there are relatively small changes in life-style that can make life worth living again. For example, spacing activities throughout the day is often necessary. Physically demanding jobs, such as gardening or housework, need to be done in small steps. Mowing the lawn and doing a number of tasks around the house in one morning will leave you exhausted and in pain. Spread the load throughout the day, or even over two days.

Home modifications

Modification of home and garden may be necessary. A chair-lift, a change of furniture or a new garden design that does not need strenuous activity to maintain it can all help. Assistance in such matters can be given by an occupational therapist, who is able to assess just what is needed and advise on suitable aids and appliances (see Chapter 8).

Many people find that after a few years their osteoarthritis settles or even becomes easier. Exceptions to this are those people who will need drugs or surgery to make life bearable. But compared with the total number of people who suffer from arthritis, these exceptions are relatively few.

Remember that the aim is to live life to the full in spite of osteoarthritis.

6

Treatment (2): the drug-free way

This chapter in some ways overlaps the previous chapter on self-help. The various specialties, such as physiotherapy and occupational therapy, are able to advise on ways of easing pain and increasing mobility without recourse to drugs or surgery. Other specialized techniques such as acupuncture, treatment by chiropractors or osteopaths can help some sufferers.

Physiotherapy

Physiotherapy is one of the first-line treatments that follows a firm diagnosis of osteoarthritis. In the UK, a series of sessions can be arranged at the local hospital or surgery by a general practitioner. Physiotherapists are experienced in advising on specific exercises to help each individual patient with painful osteoarthritis, such as exercises to help to strengthen the muscles around the knee joint if this is the joint that is mainly affected. Simple rhythmic tightening of the muscles of the thigh while seated helps to stabilize the joint as well as improving the range of movement possible. Similarly, simple gentle movements of the neck can be done at any time of the day to help relieve pain and stiffness. Advice can also be given on the best form of general exercise for each patient.

A further weapon in the armamentarium of the physiotherapist is heat. Warming up the muscles before exercise or other physio-therapy treatment improves the benefits of the exercise and ensures that weakened muscles are not overstrained. At home this can be done either with a heat lamp (be careful not to overdo the length of time this is used) or, more cheaply, by an old-fashioned warm bath.

This application of heat is mirrored in the general warming-up exercises before any considered exercise session. Warming-up exercises involve gentle stretching exercises of all parts of the body, thus putting each joint through its full range of movement as far as possible. A few strides up and down the room or garden or 'walking on the spot' increases heart rate and your breathing rate, thereby increasing the blood flow to muscles and joints.

51

Physiotherapists often also use hydrotherapy as an adjunct to treatment. In a specially designed pool, which is shallow, small in size and filled with warm water, exercise of damaged, painful joints can be easier because the buoyancy of the water counteracts gravitational pull. In this way, muscles can be strengthened by movements that are difficult or painful if performed out of the water. Then, after a few sessions, exercises can be tried out of water, often with good results.

A form of home hydrotherapy can be done by gentle exercise of muscles in a warm bath. This can in no way replace a specialized session in a hydrotherapy pool with a physiotherapist available to control the amount of exercise that each group of muscles is given. Too much exercise in the comfort of a warm bath can overstrain joints and muscles. Expert advice and help is vitally important when you are learning just how much effort needs to be put into exercise of any kind.

The Alexander technique

The Alexander technique can usefully be mentioned here. The founder of this technique, Frederick Matthias Alexander, an Australian actor, considered that many conditions, including arthritis, had their basis in poor posture. He considered the spine to be the most important part of the skeletal system. He said that if the spine is out of alignment many organs of the body will be affected. (Alexander also thought that illnesses were largely a disharmony of mental as well as the physical aspects of life. The techniques as practised by Alexander practitioners concentrate on both mental and physical aspects.)

Basically the Alexander technique teaches how to 'unlearn' bad habits relating to the skeletal system. We all tend to slouch in a chair or lie curled up in bed and, certainly as we get older, we walk with shoulders hunched and chin protruding before us. All these ingrained habits need to be corrected before good habits of standing and sitting can be learned – not an altogether easy task. In osteoarthritis, the Alexander approach is to concentrate on the general muscular co-ordination of the body without special focus on the painful arthritic part. In this way excess pressure, rigidity or collapse on to an arthritic joint is minimized. Much more can be learned about general muscle control, which can be beneficial in relieving strain on painful joints.

Pilates

The Pilates system is a somewhat similar method of balancing and controlling the muscular system of the body. Here emphasis is put on relaxation techniques as well as on specific exercises to develop and improve the inner muscular strength of the torso. Arthritis sufferers should check with their doctors before embarking on regular use of this technique. It is also important to avoid any excessive strain on muscles during an acute inflammatory stage of any rheumatic disorder.

Osteopathy and chiropractic

Along with practitioners of the Alexander technique, osteopaths and chiropractors consider that a healthy spine is necessary for a pain-free life. To this end, massage and manipulation of muscle and bone is practised. This does give some relief from the pain and stiffness of osteoarthritis. (Care must be taken, however, in an inflammatory stage of the condition. Similarly, these practices are of no benefit to inflammatory conditions such as rheumatoid arthritis. You should always tell your general practitioner, who is in charge of your overall care, about any alternative treatments that you are under-going.) Between treatments it is advised that some rest is taken. Although neither of these treatments can cure osteoarthritis, much relief can be obtained.

Osteopathy and chiropractic work in a similar fashion with minor differences in technique. Chiropractors usually advise an X-ray of the spine before therapy is begun, but osteopaths usually dispense with this visual aid to the anatomy of the spine.

Occupational therapy

Occupational therapy involves learning how to cope with what-ever degree of disability may be present as a result of the arthritis. Occupational therapists work mainly attached to hospitals, but some occupational therapists work on a community basis. Your doctor will be able to advise you as to what is available in your local community.

Occupational therapists are specialists in recommending new ways of doing the everyday tasks that can give difficulty in osteoarthritis. They are also able to advise on the many gadgets which are available to assist (see Chapter 8).

Acupuncture

Acupuncture is not a cure for arthritis, but it is used to relieve the chronic pain so often associated with this disease. Acupuncture has its basis in Chinese medicine. It is thought that 'life energy' flows along certain lines – termed 'meridians' – in our bodies. There are thought to be two components to this field energy, 'yin' and 'yang'. These two forces need to be balanced for a healthy mind and body. The insertion of very fine needles into these meridian lines are thought to free and balance these forces and allow energy to flow freely.

Exactly how acupuncture works is disputed. One theory subscribes to the gate theory of pain, which considers that pain is regulated by a 'gate' that prevents pain impulses passing along nerves. When the gate closes the pain is shut off. Acupuncture is thought to stimulate the closure of the gate. Another theory considers that stimulation of the acupuncture points releases pain-killing hormones called 'endorphins', which reduce the pain experienced. (Exercise is also thought to produce endorphins.)

Whatever the mechanism, acupuncture does seem to work for some people. Special pain clinics in the UK practise acupuncture, as do some general practitioners.

Massage

Massage is a well-known and ancient practice for relieving pain in the musculoskeletal system. This ancient art was revived as a treatment for painful muscles and joints by a Swedish masseur, Henri Ling. Once a treatment available only at special spa centres, therapeutic massage has now become part of the armamentarium of physiotherapists. A knowledge of physiology, anatomy and conditions that affect the musculoskeletal system is necessary for relief to be given to painful muscles and joints. By applying the correct pressure and movements for each patient, knotted muscles in spasm can be relaxed, so reducing the pain. (It is sad that massage has unfortunate connotations, since this form of therapy can give much relief to people with osteoarthritis.)

Transcutaneous electrical nerve stimulation (TENS)

TENS is a relatively recent method of relieving pain. It involves blocking the electronic gates (the nerve pathways to the brain) through which pain impulses pass. By the application of low-level electrical impulses, these pain gates are closed. A TENS machine passes these low-voltage, high-frequency impulses through the skin when the device is placed over the painful area. This is particularly helpful in dealing with small localized areas of pain. Further refinements on TENS are currently under way.

Any one of these therapies, or a combination, can be of much help in the relief of pain and stiffness in osteoarthritis. In conjunction with self-help activities discussed in Chapter 5, these non-drug therapies can lead to much relief. However, at times symptoms are so severe and joints so severely damaged that drugs or surgery becomes necessary.

7

Treatment (3): drugs and surgery

Drugs are powerful chemicals that work to cure a disease or to relieve its symptoms. Drug treatments in osteoarthritis aim to relieve the three main problems in this condition – pain, stiffness and immobility – but a complete cure with drugs is not yet possible. Various types of drugs are commonly used at present to control the symptoms of osteoarthritis.

Drugs used to treat osteoarthritis

Pain-killing (analgesic) drugs

There are a good many 'over-the-counter' pain-killing drugs that are familiar to many people. Pain-killing drugs are probably the most numerous type of medication on the pharmacist's shelf.

The most common pain-killing drugs are aspirin and paracetamol, either on their own or in some kind of combination with other drugs. People have their favourite pain-killing drug, but, as with every kind of drug, side effects need to be monitored carefully. Aspirin, a very useful drug for many conditions, can give rise to irritation of the lining of the stomach, causing pain and nausea, if taken continually in large enough doses. (The small dose – 75mg per day – advised for some people as a means of stopping dangerous blood clotting is unlikely to have this unwanted side effect.) Owing to this side effect, paracetamol is usually advised as the drug of choice if pain-killers will be needed for a considerable length of time. Neither aspirin nor paracetamol should be taken more often than at four-hourly intervals, and they certainly should not be continued for any length of time without medical advice. They are, however, both useful drugs for controlling a temporary exacerbation of pain. Taken before a gentle exercise session the initial pain of movement can be reduced.

Other useful analgesic drugs are those that have added codeine, such as Co-proxamol and Co-codamol (preparations that contain paracetamol plus codeine). One of the main disadvantages of the codeine component is that constipation can become an added problem. This can be overcome by regular exercise and a diet rich in fruit, vegetables and other fibre products.

Non-steroidal anti-inflammatory drugs

A further group of pain-killing drugs is available – the non-steroidal anti-inflammatory drugs (NSAIDs). These drugs are useful in controlling the pain felt as a result of the worsening of the osteoarthritis. The cyclo-oxygenase drugs – COX-1 drugs and, more recently, the COX-2 drugs – are useful in suppressing pain, but, as with all drugs, can give rise to unwanted side effects such as inflammation in the gastrointestinal tract and also possible problems if you have high blood pressure. So it is important that all drugs used on a long-term basis should be reviewed regularly, first to find out if they are still effective and second to monitor the possibility of unwanted side effects. This is of special importance in older people, who can so easily be taking several drugs regularly for various conditions.

Non-steroidal anti-inflammatory drugs are also available as gels or creams for rubbing over painful joints. These preparations can do much to relieve pain when applied to joints that are readily accessible to this form of treatment. They also have the advantage of having few, if any, side effects, such as the gastrointestinal effects that can occur when non-steroidal anti-inflammatory drugs are taken by mouth.

Muscle-relaxant drugs

One further group of drugs that can relieve pain in osteoarthritis are the muscle-relaxant drugs, of which there are many. Some of the pain of osteoarthritis arises from spasm of the muscles around the affected joint, and muscle-relaxant drugs help to reduce this painful spasm and so may allow further exercise to strengthen these muscles.

Corticosteroids

Corticosteroids are infrequently used in osteoarthritis (in direct contradistinction to rheumatoid arthritis, in which they have an important part to play). Occasionally, however, an injection of a corticosteroid drug can be given into a painful joint during an acute inflammatory phase of osteoarthritis. The effect is temporary and such treatment is recommended only in certain circumstances, such as when surgery is being awaited.

Other drugs

There are other drugs currently being researched for the treatment of osteoarthritis, including drugs that exert a protective effect on the cartilage of joints. As yet no definite conclusions have been reached, but some of the prospects show great promise.

Surgery for osteoarthritis

There are many, many people with osteoarthritis for whom non-surgical measures suffice and enable them to lead satisfactory lives. There are some people, however, who need surgery of one kind or another. The criteria for needing surgery must be evaluated for each individual patient. As a rough guide, uncontrollable pain – and especially if sleep is impossible because of pain – may point to the need for surgical intervention. Increasing immobility and the inability to attend to personal bodily functions may also require surgery. There are various surgical procedures available for specific types of disability.

Arthroscopy

Arthroscopy is the procedure by which the surgeon can see inside a joint and then carry out any necessary surgery on it. The knee is the joint most commonly operated on in this way. A small probe is inserted into the joint, and, by looking at a monitor or screen, the surgeon is able to see the exact state of the inside of the joint. This type of 'keyhole' surgery is useful in removing any loose bodies that have been broken off and are causing pain or locking of the joint. Many other minor abnormalities of the cartilage or ligaments of the knee can also be treated in this way.

Osteoarthritis is not cured by this type of surgery and careful evaluation of the symptoms need to be done before arthroscopy is recommended. Much relief can be gained, however, by the removal of any loose pieces of cartilage or bone in the joint.

This type of surgery is usually undertaken in younger people, especially in those who have had a previous injury to the knee joint. However, older people can also benefit from a general 'tidying up' of odd pieces of cartilage inside the joint while awaiting surgery for a replacement joint.

Osteotomy

Osteotomy is a surgical procedure that is of value in some, specific conditions. For example, a young person who has had a severe injury to a specific joint, such as the hip or knee, and who is in severe pain from the subsequent development of osteoarthritis may benefit from an osteotomy.

This operation involves surgically fracturing the bone below the affected joint. The bone is then realigned in a more satisfactory position to withstand the everyday stresses and strains involved in the joint. In this way the painful arthritic parts of the joint are relieved of stress. The realigned bone must be secured in position by plates and screws. Osteotomy is a major procedure but one that can be valuable as a temporary measure in young people, in whom a hip or knee replacement may not be advisable because of their age.

Arthrodesis

'Arthrodesis' means the fusion of a joint. An arthrodesis is a good way of eliminating the pain that is felt when a severely arthritic joint is moved (as it can be many times during the course of a day). However, it has its disadvantages. The joint that is operated on will be completely immovable. So, for example, an arthrodesed knee joint will result in a stiff, rigid leg that cannot be bent at all at the knee. Normal walking is therefore impossible, and difficulties can also be experienced on sitting down since the leg will be sticking out awkwardly. Again, arthrodesis is rarely done and is mainly confined to younger people who have had an injury to a joint.

Joint replacement surgery

Joint replacement is by far the most common procedure available today for severely arthritic knees and hips. These operations have been one of the major advances in surgery over recent years, largely owing to the availability of suitable materials for making the replacement joints as well as advances in surgical technique.

Hip replacement surgery

It was in the 1950s that the currently used technique of hip replacement was first established. The two separate parts of the joint being replaced are made of two different types of material – the thigh bone end of the joint is made of titanium or stainless steel and the pelvic part is made of a polyethylene compound. A brief word about the anatomy of the hip joint will clarify what is being done. The hip joint is a 'ball-and-socket' joint. The 'ball', which is the rounded end of the thigh bone (femur), fits neatly into the 'socket', which is the acetabulum on the outside of the pelvic bone (see Figure 3).

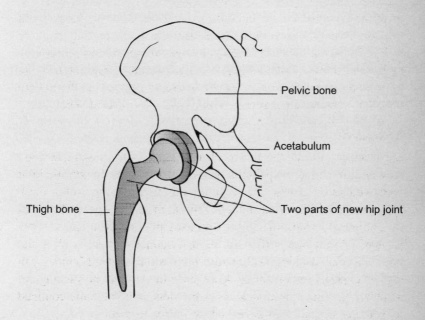

Figure 3 A hip replacement

Replaced joints do not last for ever, as Melanie's case history shows. Although further replacements can be done, they are sometimes not as successful as the original replacement. It is this fact that makes joint replacements inadvisable in younger people. On average 10–15 years is the life of a replacement joint.

Recently, a new operation, in which the ends of the bones of the affected hip joint are 're-surfaced' rather then being replaced altogether, has been tried. This technique may well be of advantage to younger people who are in need of hip surgery, but long-term effects will need to be further researched.

The pain in Melanie's hip was getting worse by the day. Her athletic prowess in younger days was finally catching up with her, and she was still only in her early forties.

She had followed all the medical and physiotherapy advice given her over the preceding four or five years when the pain had been steadily worsening, but now she had to resort to pain-killers more and more frequently. A hip replacement had been discussed a few years previously with an orthopaedic surgeon. He, however, was reluctant to do this operation in such a relatively young woman. 'You'll be needing a further replacement, Mrs Saunders, by the time you are 60 if we give you a new one now,' had been his verdict at Melanie's last visit.

That evening, when her two girls, by then aged seven and nine, were in bed, Melanie told her husband of the consultant's words. 'But I'm finding it difficult to keep up with the girls, Ken,' she confided. 'Even an easy game of tennis with them crippled me the other day. I shall be useless in walking and playing tennis and other sports soon. And I do so want to help them enjoy all the sport I enjoyed when I was their age.'

Six months later, Melanie again sat in the orthopaedic consulting room. Her stick, which she now found indispensable, lay awkwardly on the floor at her feet. The conversation had followed much the same lines as before, but now there seemed a greater need to pursue the possibility of a hip replacement. 'You see, I would rather be able to enjoy the next ten years or so with my daughters, even if it means further surgery when I get older.

So, if it is possible, I would rather have a new hip now than wait any longer.'

In view of the rapid deterioration of Melanie's hip the wait for surgery was only a few months. All went well with the operation and Melanie scrupulously followed all the advice that she was given on exercise and rest. Within six months she was able to join in with many of her daughters' sporting activities, giving them her experience of sport of all kinds.

But time passes. Both girls are now married and one is expecting her first child – and Melanie was once more in a good deal of pain. It seemed just like a re-run of her previous discussions with the orthopaedic surgeon, who is now about to retire. 'Do you regret your decision, Melanie, to have a new hip in your forties?' he asked. 'Because you realize that we will now have to replace it.'

'I knew this would come eventually,' Melanie replied, 'but I really have no regrets. I've thoroughly enjoyed the past 15 years with my daughters and being able to look after the family properly.'

Melanie's second hip replacement was difficult and it took her many more weeks to return to a normal lifestyle than it had done after her first operation. But today she is striding around the village with her new granddaughter as if she were once again in her forties.

Knee replacement surgery

The knee is the second most commonly replaced joint in osteoarthritis. The knee is a complex joint, involving not only the movements of bending and straightening but also small, but vital, movements of rotation. These movements involve specific ligaments inside the joint known as the cruciate ligaments. Replacement of the knee joint is done either with or without replacement of these ligaments, depending on the amount of disease that is present.

As with the hip joint the two new parts of the joint are made of different materials. The upper part of the joint is made of metal, which is placed over the lower end of the thigh bone (femur). A plastic material is attached to the upper end of the shin bone (tibia).

Most knee replacements will function satisfactorily for around 15 years. So, once again, it is not a good idea to replace a knee joint in a young person unless absolutely necessary.

What happens before joint replacement surgery?
It is usual for the pre-surgery assessment to be done a few days before your admission to the hospital ward for surgery. In this way all the necessary information about your general health is obtained. Any problem can be found and dealt with and so valuable time on the ward before surgery is not lost. Also, at this time blood may be taken and stored in case it is needed during or after the operation for a blood transfusion. In this way the patient's own blood can be used. Some of the tests that may be done on this routine pre-surgery assessment are:

• a blood test, to determine if there is any anaemia and to check on the levels of normal chemicals in the blood, to determine the blood group in case you need a blood transfusion at a later date and to store a couple of units of blood in case you need a blood transfusion during or after the operation;
• a urine test, to check that there is no infection in the urinary tract;
• an electrocardiogram (ECG), to make sure that the heart is functioning normally (if any abnormality is found the anaesthetic may need to be adjusted);
• a chest X-ray, to make sure that no chest infection or other abnormality is present (again, if any abnormality is found the anaesthetic may need to be adjusted); and
• an X-ray of the joint to be operated on so that the surgeon can see its exact state.

The results of all these tests will be added to the medical notes before you are admitted to hospital for surgery.

Optimizing recovery from surgery
During the period between deciding that an operation is necessary and the actual surgery (which is sometimes a long time), there are things that you can do that will help in your eventual recovery.

Weight control is all important, so if this is a factor for you it is well worth trying to lose a few pounds. Excess weight means that the surgery itself can be more difficult, and this can cause extra, unnecessary bleeding. Overweight also usually implies that breathing is not as effective as it might be, and this in turn will mean that extra care needs to be taken with the anaesthetic. After the operation, excess weight will mean extra strain on the new joint.

Any physical problem with the heart, the lungs or any other system of the body needs to be adequately treated. Also, of course, you must be sure that the surgeon, anaesthetist and hospital staff are aware of any other medical condition and any drugs that you are taking. Most wards will ask for a sample of the drugs you take regularly to be brought in on the day of admission.

If you smoke, try to stop or at least to cut down. Healthy lungs will take to an anaesthetic more readily. Remember, too, that hospitals are definitely no-smoking areas, so you will not be able to smoke at all during your stay. So be ahead of the game and stop smoking long before your surgery.

Keep as fit as possible in the run-up to surgery. A good diet and as much exercise as you can manage will be a bonus when it comes to post-operative recovery. Remember that even if your lower limbs are not too good on the exercise front, upper limb exercises can do much for future muscle tone and better breathing after surgery.

After surgery

After a hip replacement
It is usual to have complete bed-rest for one or two days after a hip replacement. A triangular-shaped cushion will be placed between the thighs. This ensures that the new hip is kept in the correct position while healing takes place.

Physiotherapy from an early stage is an important part of post-operative care. This ensures that muscles are kept in trim as well as teaching movements that are safe. Gentle exercise also reduces the risk of a blood clot in the leg veins; elastic stockings are also worn to assist in preventing this complication.

Initially, after a day or two, you will start walking with the aid of a walking frame. Following on from this, it is amazing how quickly people progress to normal walking, first of all with crutches and then with walking sticks. Pain-free movement will seem a miracle once the discomforts of the operation are over.

The hospital stay is usually about seven or ten days. Care will need to be taken at home for a further six weeks. Physiotherapy will need to be continued, as will normal walking activities. Hydrotherapy after a few weeks will also be found to be helpful in strengthening weakened muscles.

After a knee replacement

After a knee replacement, rehabilitation using the new joint is begun early. In some hospitals physiotherapy is started on the first day after the operation with the use of a machine that moves the knee joint passively for several hours at a time. Walking is also started early with the aid of a walking frame at first, progressing to crutches and finally to a walking stick. Again progress can be rapid when it is realized that there is no longer any arthritic pain in the joint when it is moved.

General considerations after joint replacement surgery

Continuing gentle exercise is important. Exercises advised by the physiotherapist can easily become part of the daily routine when you return home. Walking, slowly at first and gradually increasing the speed and distance, is an excellent way to continue rehabilitation.

Car driving is not advisable for the first two or three months after hip surgery. Being a passenger in a car before this time will need special care in getting in and out of the vehicle. The leg that has been operated on needs to be kept as straight as possible during the early stages. This can be achieved in these circumstances by sitting as far back into the car seat as possible before swinging the leg in.

Bathing also needs care. Be sure that there is someone readily available at first to give help if necessary. A bath seat is useful initially as are hand rails on the sides of the bath. If you have had a hip replacement, keep the operated leg as straight as possible and avoid pivoting on the hip.

Low seats on chairs and toilets are to be avoided as far as possible. Have a high seat added to the toilet seat and make sure that chairs have supporting arms to help you to get up. Again, keep the operated leg – if it is the hip that has been replaced – as straight as possible.

Avoid bending. Do not pick anything up from the floor initially, and get help with the putting on of shoes and socks in the early days.

There are mechanical aids for this activity if you live alone (see Chapter 8).

Avoid weight gain. Your new hip or knee will not take kindly to extra weight, so keep up the diet and the gentle exercise.

If care is taken for three to four months after joint replacement surgery, results are generally excellent. The quality of life is vastly improved by the surgery and should continue to be so for up to 15 years. After this time it is possible that further surgery will be required – at least pending further research into other types of surgery.

8
Aids and appliances

The number of aids and appliances available to help with the difficulties in daily living with osteoarthritis seems to proliferate daily. Only a small sample of them is suggested here. For a wider selection, contact either the Disabled Living Foundation (see page 82) or the Mobility Information Services (see page 82). In the UK, help can also be found from the local branch of Social Services. Your general practitioner will be able to put you in contact and also suggest the type of aid that would be most helpful in each individual case. Following on from this will be a visit from an occupational therapist and a member of the Social Services team. Your specific needs will be assessed and suggestions will be made as to which aid would be of most help. This may mean that certain adaptations to your home will need to be done, ranging from a downstairs bathroom or a stair lift to more mundane things such as grab rails on each side of the toilet and bath or advice on how to cope more easily with tasks in the kitchen.

Financial help may be available for the more major changes through a disabled facilities grant – this will be means-tested. The more minor items, such as grab rails, are usually fitted free of charge.

Aids available for osteoarthritis of the hip, knee, back and neck

Both pain and stiffness can make for difficulty in performing everyday tasks. Fortunately there is much that can help with both these symptoms. (And do remember that exercise of any kind, if undertaken gently, is good for arthritis. As long as regular rest periods are included in the daily timetable, general household tasks can be beneficial.)

Aids to general living
Aids to general living include:

- long-handled pick-up tongs to retrieve objects from the floor (these can also be used – carefully! – to reach objects on high shelves);
- special electric plugs with extra-large push-in knobs for electrical appliances;
- light-weight carpet sweepers (to replace your heavy vacuum cleaner);
- a suitably comfortable chair.

Indeed, such a chair is a 'must' for any arthritis sufferer. The seat should be as high as possible – allowing the feet to touch the floor when seated – for ease of getting up. Arms should be at the right height and be able to be grasped firmly – polished wood in this situation can be dangerous. There should be a good support for the back and the neck. If disability is severe, there are chairs available in which the seat moves upwards when activated by a button. This will help with the sometimes difficult task of getting up from sitting. It will be necessary to try different types of chairs before a suitable one is found. Remember that you will probably be sitting in the chair for many hours over the day, so do be sure that your money is well spent. (There is a booklet available from the Arthritis Research Campaign (see page 81) entitled 'Are You Sitting Comfortably?', which gives excellent advice on choosing a suitable chair.)

Aids in the bedroom

Aids in the bedroom include:

- a firm comfortable mattress, which is vital, and choosing one should not be hurried;
- duvets, which are more convenient than blankets and sheets and which help to make making the bed easier.

Aids in the bathroom

Aids in the bathroom include:

- hand rails for getting down on to the toilet and rising up off it – these are a necessity and they should be securely fixed and maintained in the correct position;

- a foot-operated flushing system;
- hand rails on either side of the bath (although many people with arthritis find a shower easier to manage than a bath);
- bath seats of several different types; and
- special seats for use in the shower.

Aids for outside the home and for hobbies

It is important that outside interests should be kept up. As mentioned previously it is all too easy to fall into a depressed state if hobbies and interests have to be given up. Again, however, there are aids that can assist with a variety of hobbies.

For gardening:

- long-handled shears, forks, rakes and hoes are available in light-weight materials, which can make many of the routine gardening jobs easier;
- flower beds can be raised so that kneeling or stooping is unnecessary; and
- light-weight seats for planting or weeding in the raised beds are also useful.

Many of these specialized tools can be found in ordinary garden centres as well as in centres for disabled living.

For sewing and other handicrafts:

- needle threaders are a boon to osteoarthritic hands – there are several varieties available, and some are very easy to use; any good sewing or craft shop should be able to offer a choice;
- special easily opening scissors are available; and
- small ironing boards suitable for putting on a table top will be helpful in pressing small areas of stitching.

Car driving is still possible for most people with osteoarthritis and can be a mobility boon. Here again there are a number of aids available:

- a car with automatic drive would be a major expense, but the constant changing of gears with much use of the left hand and foot is eliminated (a different type of driving technique has to be learnt, but many people would never change back to a manual car once they had got used to an automatic car);

- power steering is common in modern cars and does much to relieve strain on the neck and shoulders; and
- wide-angled driving mirrors can also be helpful in that there is less twisting to be done when reversing; again this will take a while to become used to.

Aids available for osteoarthritis of the hands

Heberden's nodes of the fingers are more of a nuisance than a cause of actual disability. However, the combination of Heberden's nodes and osteoarthritis of the thumb joint can cause much disability when small intricate tasks are being performed with the hands. As well as pain and stiffness there can also be some weakness of grip. Therefore the ability to cope with household and everyday tasks can become somewhat limited. There are a number of aids that can assist.

Aids in the kitchen

Various aids are available for use in the kitchen. Opening tins can be difficult. There are several kinds of aid, from mats that keep the tin stable while it is being opened to electric tin openers (which can also be attached to the wall). All of these can help. Opening jars can also be difficult (and not only for people with arthritis!). A plastic or rubber cap that increases the purchase that can be exerted on the lid of the jar is a simple solution. There is also a device that fits under a shelf and so allows a two-handed grip to be used when opening jars.

For cutting and chopping foods, a spiked surface will hold the food steady while it is being prepared. This works with all types of foods. In addition, working surfaces should be as large as possible and free from too much equipment. A big, free surface allows for easier movement without the need to lift heavy pans and dishes.

Taps that need a screwing action to turn them on can cause problems. If at all possible, change your taps to the lever-type tap. However, this can be expensive, and there are tap-turning devices that fit loosely over a standard screw tap.

A microwave is a good investment since microwave cooking can avoid the need to lift heavy saucepans. They are also very much easier to keep clean than a conventional oven. Cookers, whether electric or gas, can be adapted, for example, to have bigger, more easily controllable knobs. The appropriate electricity or gas companies can give advice and help on this aspect. A trolley is useful for transporting food into other rooms.

Aids in the bedroom and bathroom

Some aspects of dressing can be a problem if osteoarthritis of the hands is severe. A few aids will make life easier:

- Velcro fastenings on coats and dresses can sometimes take the place of buttons, but, alternatively, if buttons are necessary, there are button hooks available to cope with these;
- bras that are either slip-on or that have a front fastening are helpful;
- slip-on shoes or those with a Velcro fastening instead of buckles and laces can be helpful while shoe horns, and devices for pulling on socks, may also be useful.

Washing can also give rise to difficulties if the hands are badly affected by osteoarthritis. In addition to the aids mentioned above, there are several others that may help:

- 'soap on a rope', which will prevent the soap slipping away;
- washing mitts or gloves; and
- long-handled loofahs or brushes.

Just a few of the aids and appliances that are available are described above. Many more can be found by either visiting one of the disabled living centres or writing to one of the groups concerned with the care of people with arthritis. The addresses of these are to be found on pages 81–82.

A final word

A diagnosis of osteoarthritis is not the end of the world. As we have already seen, osteoarthritis is not a fatal disease. It is one that has its 'ups and downs'. Fortunately osteoarthritis often seems to settle down into a pattern with which the sufferer is able to live successfully – even though perhaps only after a joint replacement or some changes in lifestyle.

Self-help measures, drugs and surgery all play their part in achieving this end, and each person has his or her own favourite way of coping. But above all it is important that spirits are kept up on a daily basis. It may be that extensive pain-free walks, participation in a previously enjoyed sport or even climbing stairs with ease are no longer possibilities. However, efforts to compensate for changes in lifestyle by taking an interest in more suitable activities will do much to keep depressive feelings at bay. 'Easier said than done' possibly, but nevertheless well worth working at.

It must also be realized that tasks previously undertaken, and finished, in a relatively short time span can no longer be achieved so quickly. Sensible spacing of daily chores so as to minimize fatigue and a worsening of pain must be seen as a priority. Putting some gentle exercise into the daily timetable will also give relief, however tedious this may seem at first. Remember that immobility is to be avoided at all costs – and this goal is possible for the vast majority of people with osteoarthritis.

Life with osteoarthritis is not easy to begin with. However, with a positive outlook and genuine efforts to reduce its effects, the aim of living life to the full with osteoarthritis can be attained.

Glossary

Acromegaly	A disease characterized by the overgrowth of bone
Acute	Describes a disease or condition that arises quickly and lasts a short time
Aerobic exercise	Exercise that strengthens the heart and lungs by increasing oxygen consumption
Analgesic	Pain-killing drug
Aneurysm	Ballooning of a blood vessel
Arthralgia	Joint pain
Arthroplasty	Complete joint replacement
Arthroscopy	Optical visualization of the inside of a joint
Aspirin	An *analgesic*. Has other uses, such as a small daily dose that reduces the possibility of blood clots. Also reduces fever
Baker's cyst	Swelling at back of knee filled with *synovial fluid* from a tear in the capsule of the joint
Boucher's disease	Osteoarthritis of the thumb joint
Bursa	Fibrous sac lined with synovial tissue
Cartilage	A dense connective tissue of which there are several types, one of which lines the ends of bones in a joint and is affected in osteoarthritis
Cervical spine	Bones making up the neck region of the spine, of which there are seven
Chronic	Describes a disease or condition that persists over a long time
Crepitus	Creaking sound in diseased joints

77

Effusion	Collection of fluid (for example, inside a joint)
Endorphins	Chemicals in the body that have pain-relieving properties
Enzymes	Catalysts that start off chemical reactions in the body
Fibromyalgia	Condition in which the muscles are painful and tender
Gout	Painful condition of joint caused by an excess of uric acid crystals
Heberden's nodes	Arthritic swellings on the joints of the fingers
Isotope scanning	Imaging conducted after a substance has been injected into the bloodstream to show up any abnormalities
Ligament	Strong band of fibrous tissue found especially around joints that, together with attached muscles, hold the joints in place
Loose bodies	Small pieces of bone or *cartilage* that have broken off from inside the joint; the main cause of 'locked' joints
Lyme disease	A disease transmitted by ticks with arthritis as part of the symptoms
Occupational therapist	Specialist giving advice on equipment and on how to minimize disability caused by disease
Orthopaedic surgeon	Doctor specializing in conditions affecting the skeleton
Osteopath	Practitioner specializing in disorders of the skeleton, who considers that many disorders are due to malalignment of the spine
Osteophyte	Bony outgrowth occurring near areas of damaged *cartilage* inside a joint. These can break off and form '*loose bodies*'

Osteoporosis	Condition in which there is a thinning and weakening of bones, usually found in middle-aged and elderly women
Physiotherapist	Practitioner who employs physical methods of pain relief such as heat and manipulation. Also aids breathing after surgery
Polymyalgia rheumatica	Disease causing pain and stiffness in thighs, shoulders and neck. Affects the elderly and is treated with corticosteroids
Prednisolone	Corticosteroid drug used to treat some arthritic diseases, mainly rheumatoid arthritis and *polymyalgia rheumatica*
Psoriasis	Skin disease that can have arthritis as one of the symptoms
Rheumatologist	Doctor specializing in the whole range of rheumatic disorders
Sprain	Tear, or excessive stretching, of a *ligament*, as when the ankle is forcibly twisted
Stenosis	Narrowing of space inside a bony structure such as the spine
Synovial fluid	Clear sticky fluid that 'oils' some joints
Synovial membrane	Membrane lining the capsule of specific joints; it produces *synovial fluid*, which lubricates the joint

Useful addresses

Arthritis Care
18–20 Stephenson Way
London NW1 2HD
Tel: (020) 7380 6500
Helpline: (0808) 800 4050
Website: www.arthritiscare.org.uk

Arthritis Research Campaign (ARC)
PO Box 177
Chesterfield
Derbyshire S41 7TQ
Tel: (01246) 558033
Website: www.arc.org.uk

British Acupuncture Council
Park House
63 Jeddo Road
London W12 9HQ
Tel: (020) 8735 0400

British Association of Occupational Therapists
106–114 Borough High Street
London SE1 1LB
Tel: (020) 7357 6480

Chartered Society of Physiotherapy
14 Bedford Row
London WC1R 4ED
Tel: (020) 7306 6666